EVERYDAY DETOX

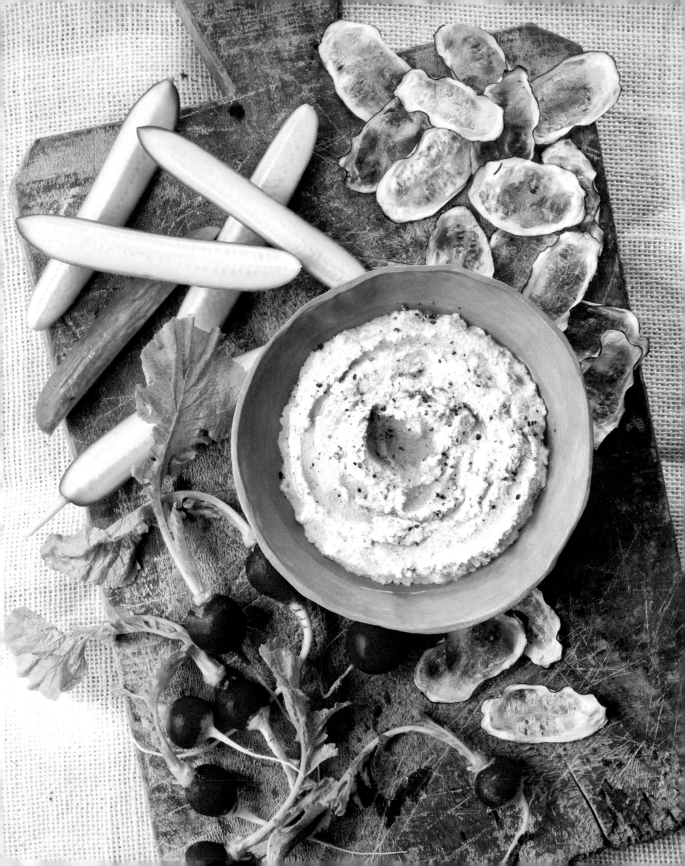

EVERYDAY
DETOX

100 Easy Recipes to Remove Toxins,
Promote Gut Health, and Lose Weight Naturally

MEGAN GILMORE

PHOTOGRAPHY BY NICOLE FRANZEN

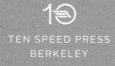

TEN SPEED PRESS
BERKELEY

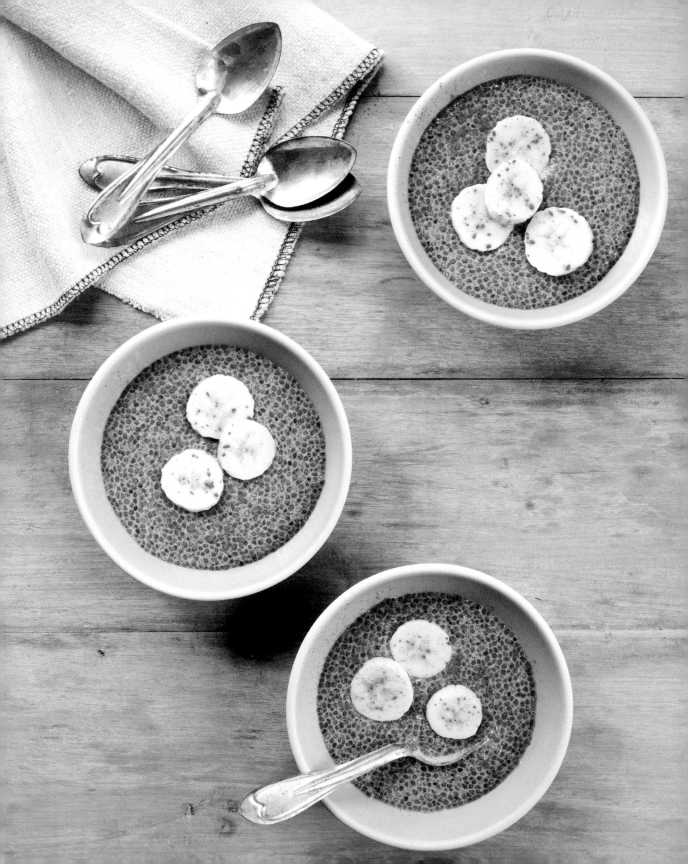

To my husband, Austin, and our adorable son,
my captive taste testers and the loves of my life.

contents

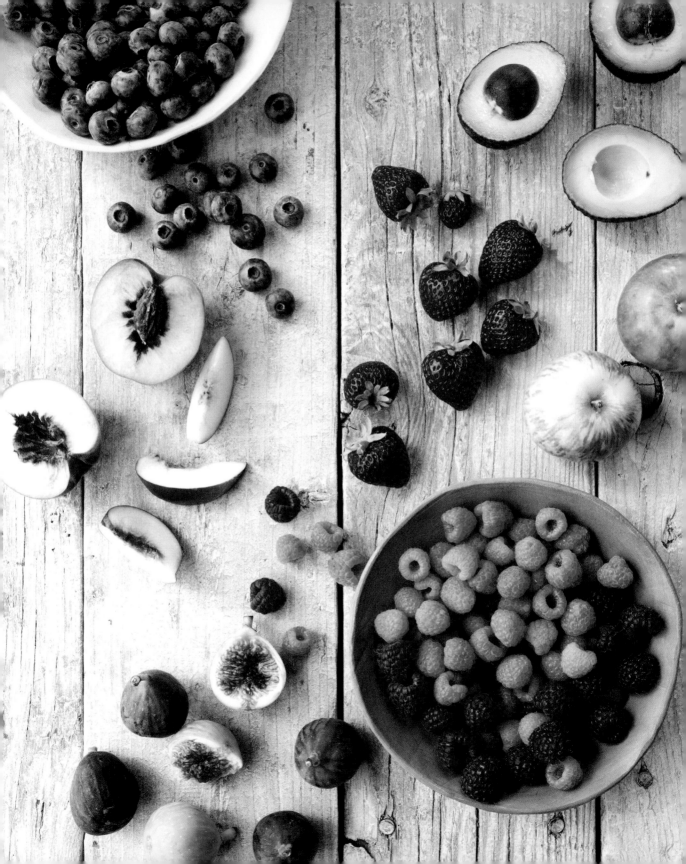

introduction

The nutrition world can be daunting. With all of the hype surrounding the latest celebrity diets and weight-loss products, we are bombarded daily with conflicting health news—leaving us generally baffled about what to eat.

Instead of looking to the next diet trend for the answer to effortless weight loss and lasting health, let's focus on what we know really works: eating whole foods. Consistently eating real, unprocessed foods is the key to naturally detoxifying and uncovering the body you've always desired. The recipes in this book will help you do just that, as they have been strategically developed with whole foods to help you reach your health goals. You'll be eating well year-round, without giving up any of the favorite dishes that you love.

That's what's special about this "everyday" approach to detox—instead of taking drastic measures, you'll be enjoying delicious meals made from whole foods on a regular basis. The following recipes will help optimize your digestion, gently remove toxins from your body, and soon have you looking and feeling better than ever before. You'll have no problem dropping those few extra pounds, because you'll be eating clean and healthy meals every day—with room for treats. Best of all, you'll achieve the results you want by simply making a few swaps in your pantry and using better ingredients to make your favorite dishes. No calorie counting or juice fasting required.

MY STORY

It might surprise you to hear that I wasn't raised as a healthy eater. Quite the contrary, in fact! Growing up in a military family, we moved often and relied heavily on packaged convenience foods and drive-through windows. I was accustomed to having many of my meals "super-sized" and thought that a glass of skim milk mixed with a package of chocolate breakfast powder was a complete and healthy breakfast.

Despite my typical diet of highly processed meals, my interest in preparing food started at a young age. One of my earliest creations in the kitchen was my own take on "cheesecake," which featured a slice of Wonder Bread topped with a thick layer of margarine, processed cheese, white sugar, and a dash of colored sprinkles for good measure. Sounds appealing, right? I was so proud that I couldn't wait to share it with my family. My parents, supportive as always, were brave enough to take a bite . . . but they never bought sprinkles again.

I still enjoy sharing my kitchen creations with my friends and family, but luckily for all of us, my ingredients and taste buds have improved over the years. I've traded in refined sugars and processed dairy substitutes for their all-natural counterparts, without giving up any of my favorite dishes. Not only do these higher quality ingredients make my meals healthier, but they tend to make them taste better, too.

Of course, this change didn't happen overnight. My steady diet of refined sugar and greasy meals continued well into my college years—where I finally got my wake-up call. I suddenly found myself feeling bloated, sluggish, and stuck with a closet full of clothes that no longer fit. My poor eating habits, paired with a hefty class load and reduced activity level, had finally caught up with me. This is when my interest in health and nutrition began. It was inadvertently sparked by a vain desire to get my closet back.

Influenced by fitness magazines and college friends, I embarked on a calorie-counting regimen that would soon leave me feeling famished and frazzled. While I did lose some weight, I also found myself becoming obsessed with thoughts of food and calories all day long. Eating was no longer a pleasure, but an exhausting exercise in willpower and number crunching. Despite my best efforts, I could never stick to a strict calorie limit for long before giving in to the urge to binge. This led to feelings of failure and a resolve to "make up" for my transgressions the next day with an even stricter diet. Thus began my pattern of yo-yo dieting—something I'd struggle with through the rest of college and beyond.

Over the next few years, I ate my way through a series of diets, including low-carb, low-fat, raw food, and vegan, hoping I'd eventually find the "magic solution" to my weight problems. However, no matter which approach I tried, none of them gave me the lasting results I was looking for.

What I realized after all of these failed diet attempts was that they didn't work for me because I was approaching them with an all-or-nothing mentality. I was either on a diet, or I wasn't—and when I fell off the wagon, I fell off big time. (Usually into a large pile of potato chips and chocolate chip cookies.) This cycle of bingeing and restriction took quite a toll on my body, leaving me with more wrinkles and cellulite than anyone my age should have accumulated. What had started as a vain attempt to lose weight had actually left me looking and feeling worse than ever.

It wasn't until I ditched all of the drastic diets that I finally saw results. The key to healing my body and getting past this cycle of yo-yo dieting was to change the quality of the foods I ate, and how I ate them, rather than radically giving up an entire food group or setting unrealistic calorie goals. I learned that, just like a pendulum, the more severe an approach goes in one direction, like committing to a strict diet, the more drastically it will eventually swing back in the other direction, turning into an all-out binge session. By making gradual and manageable changes, I finally set myself up to succeed.

For me, those gradual changes started in the kitchen. My passion for cooking was as strong as ever, but this time I chose to place my focus on making delicious meals using real, whole food ingredients. This is where my previous junk food habits and picky palate came in handy. I was able to re-create my old favorites, without making them taste too "healthy." By allowing myself all of the comfort foods and sweets that I wanted—just made with upgraded ingredients—I felt both physically and emotionally satisfied and finally happy with how my clothes fit again!

With a renewed passion for nutrition and health, along with a desire to help others, I attended the Institute of Integrative Nutrition to become a holistic health coach, and was later certified in clinical nutrition through NHI College. This education has equipped me with broad insight into nutrition and preventive care, with a focus on holistic nutrition and practical lifestyle management techniques. I also trained with fellow clinical nutritionist and detox expert Natalia Rose, who provided me with a fresh perspective on not only what to eat, but also how to eat it. Armed with this new knowledge, I wanted to share it with the world.

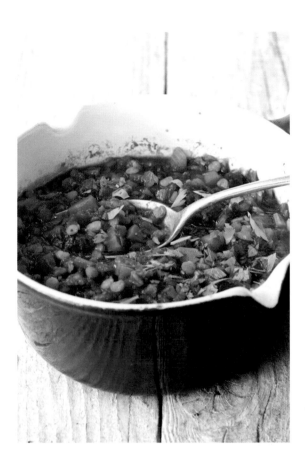

Today, I share my recipes and healthy living tips at Detoxinista.com, in the hopes that my own experience can help others who have struggled with dieting and healthy-living challenges. (To see more photos of recipes in this book, visit Detoxinista.com/cookbook.) While there is quite a bit of conflicting nutritional advice floating around, the one thing that most experts seem to agree on is that eating more whole foods and less processed ones is a step in the right direction. This is the concept that underlies all of my recipes, so I hope that you'll enjoy them as much as my family does!

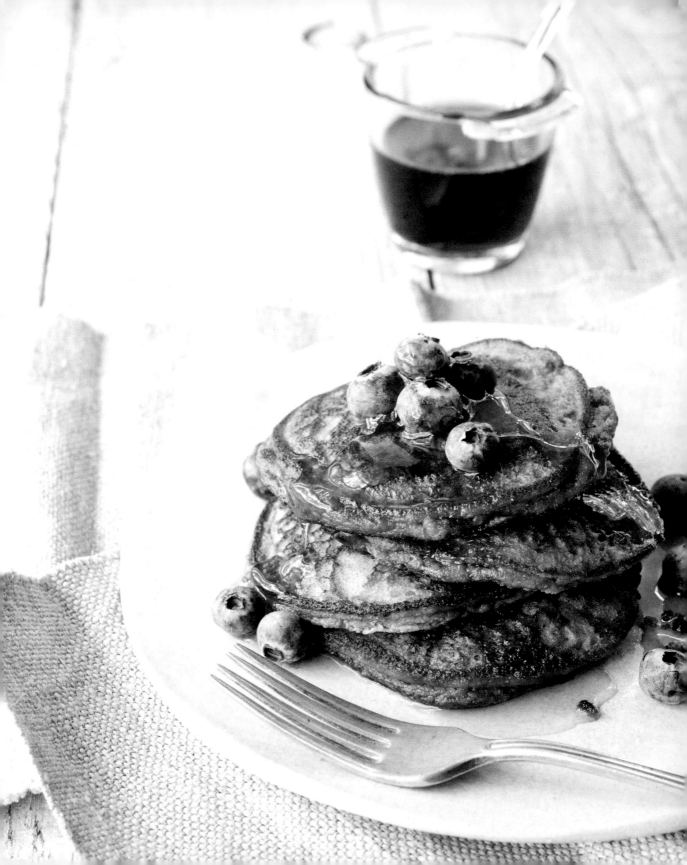

an easy approach
to detoxing

The term *detox* is often associated with fad diets and quick-fix schemes, but it doesn't have to refer to something so drastic. In fact, I think you'll find my flexible approach to detoxing quite easy and delicious.

By definition, a detox is simply a method of ridding the body of poisonous substances—not just addictive ones, such as drugs and alcohol, but also processed foods, refined sugars, and chemical additives that aren't fit for human consumption. Packaged foods, loaded with vague additives and chemical preservatives that are intended to give them the most attractive color, taste, and texture possible, now fill up the majority of our supermarket shelves. Certain manufacturers have even gone to great lengths to develop the perfect ratio of sugar, fat, and salt to make their products irresistible and downright addictive. If you've ever tried to stop at just one potato chip, you know they're on to something.

Not only are these packaged foods loaded with preservatives and chemicals, but the packaging itself may also pose a risk to our health. The petrochemical bisphenol A (commonly known as BPA), often found in plastic water bottles and canned food linings, has been shown to increase a person's risk of cardiovascular disease and diabetes, according to a study published in *The Journal of the American Medical Association*.[1] You'll notice that fresh, whole foods are rarely sold in a package, so by simply avoiding packaged convenience foods, you'll be making a positive impact on your health—without even changing how much or how often you eat.

Eating fresh, whole foods also means you can stop crunching numbers every time you're ready to pick up your fork. Calorie counting has become a popular practice but is a flawed approach because it doesn't take into account the quality of the foods we're consuming nor the body's ability to digest natural foods versus processed ones. While a 100-calorie package of cookies might have the same number of calories as an apple, the fresh fruit will provide significantly more nutrients, along with enzymes and fiber, making it much more likely to keep us satisfied until our next meal. On the other hand, when we eat foods that are high in calories but low in nutrients, we're more likely to feel hungry and deprived, leading to overeating and an endless cycle of yo-yo dieting.

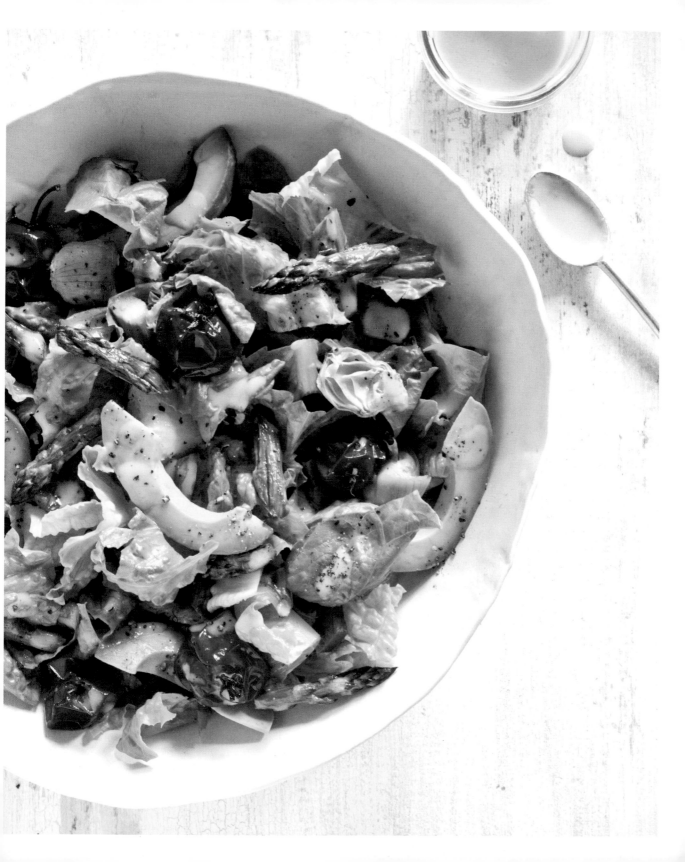

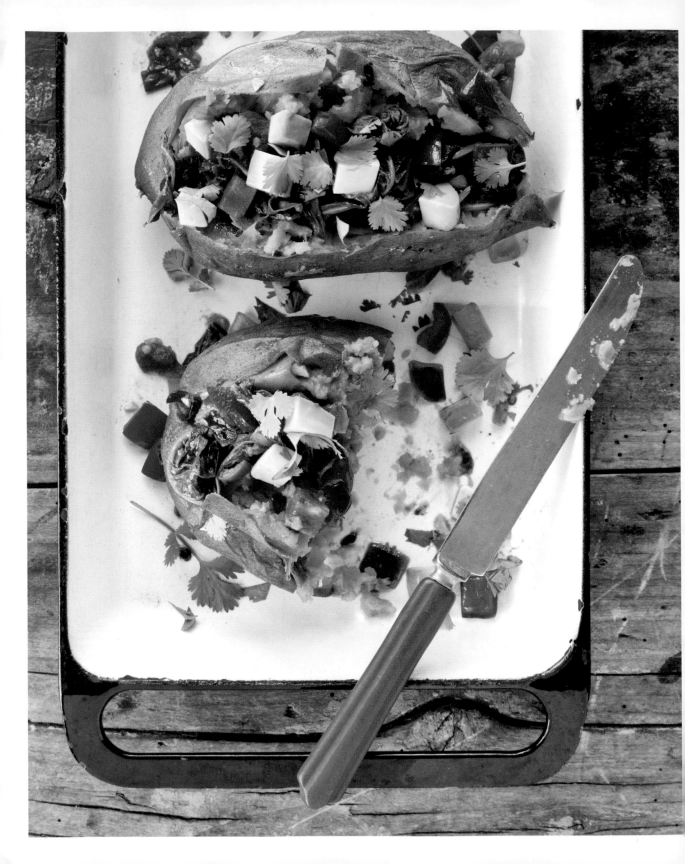

Instead of looking at the calorie count the next time you make a food choice, try thinking about where that food comes from. Is it in its natural state? How many ingredients does it contain? Do you recognize all of those ingredients? Better yet, choose a food without a label at all. By adapting a diet rich in fresh foods, you'll soon find yourself naturally satisfied, eating hearty portions, and maintaining your ideal weight—without the need for a calculator.

In fact, the old concept that weight gain is simply a matter of calories in versus calories out is proving to be far from the whole story. Exposure to toxins can actually prompt weight gain, regardless of calorie intake or exercise. For example, a study published in the *Journal of Medical Toxicology* showed that rats exposed to insecticides gained weight without increased caloric intake or decreased exercise. In just four months, these rats experienced a significant increase in body fat when compared to rats not exposed to the same toxic chemicals.[2] It has also been documented that exposure to arsenic, which is routinely fed to poultry as a way to reduce infection and create an appealing pink flesh color, increases the risk of type 2 diabetes,[3] which is another factor attributed to the obesity epidemic. This is why preparing our own meals from scratch, using organic ingredients as often as possible, is more important than ever. Our health depends on it!

Luckily, by consuming less processed and factory-farmed foods and replacing them with high-quality whole food options, you'll greatly reduce your exposure to these toxic substances without sacrificing the flavors and textures that you enjoy. In effect, you'll be detoxing your body year-round, without taking any drastic measures.

To aid in the process, this book features crowd-pleasing recipes made from all-natural ingredients, so you'll avoid any feelings of deprivation while you make the transition. They've also been developed with optimal digestion in mind, to give you the most pleasurable eating experience possible—because no one wants to feel bloated or uncomfortable after a delicious meal.

THE KEY TO BETTER DIGESTION

You're about to learn the little-known secret to eating that will boost your energy, clear your skin, improve your sleep quality, and help you lose weight and keep it off! The core of this secret starts with your digestion.

Did you know that digesting food requires more energy than any other function in the human body? It's no wonder we're exhausted after a big lunch! It stands to reason, then, that the best way to free up some extra energy is to make our digestion as quick and efficient as possible. This extra energy can better support the body's other crucial functions, like circulation, respiration, and excretion, all of which help improve your complexion, oxygenate your cells, and eliminate excess waste in the body. The less waste that's stored in your body, the better you'll look and feel.

The easiest way to get started is to change the way we approach our meals. By simply adjusting how we eat, we can improve our digestion and enjoy effortless weight loss, without giving up any of the foods we love. In other words, you can still eat practically anything and everything you want—just not necessarily all at the same time. Sounds reasonable enough, right?

The following food-combining principles are key to your success. Though they may not come naturally to you at first, with just a bit of practice, eating this way will become second nature and everyone will want to know your secret.

First, let's focus on these four basic food categories:

FRESH FRUIT   STARCHES   ANIMAL PROTEIN   NUTS, SEEDS &
                                                               DRIED FRUIT

With just a few exceptions, the goal for optimal digestion is to *not* mix these categories together in the same meal. This simplified approach is closer to the diet of our ancestors, who ate just one or two foods at a time as they came across them in nature. They would have to hunt and gather for several more hours before moving on to their next meal. Clearly, a steak-and-potato dinner wouldn't be very likely for a caveman. It wasn't until the advent of agriculture, along with improved food transportation and storage, that our meals became much more complicated and difficult to digest.

What can you enjoy along with one of these categories? All-you-can-eat vegetables. Nonstarchy vegetables, such as zucchini, broccoli, cauliflower, carrots, cabbage, onions, collard greens, green beans, and more are all easily broken down in the stomach, so they are considered neutral for our purposes. This means you can eat them anytime with anything. Any vegetable that can be eaten raw can be considered nonstarchy, though you are welcome to enjoy them cooked, too. Other all-natural additions, such as butter and cold-pressed oils, nondairy milks, honey, pure maple syrup, cocoa, and a wide range of herbs and seasonings, are also considered neutral and will provide all of the flavors you need to create delectable, crowd-pleasing dishes.

I realize that this approach to eating goes against much of the mainstream mind-set, in which a balanced meal consists of a serving of complex carbs, protein, and fat at each sitting, but have you ever thought about what these types of meals do to our digestive system? The production of hydrochloric acid, which is necessary for digesting protein, is hindered by the presence of starches and sugars in the stomach.[4] Insufficient hydrochloric acid can delay the whole digestive process, because it isn't until the contents of the stomach reach a highly acidic pH level that they are released into the small intestine, continuing the digestive process where most of the nutrients are absorbed.[5] The longer this undigested food remains in your stomach, the more likely it is to rot and ferment, providing a potential feeding ground for harmful yeast and bacteria. These microbes can contribute to sugar cravings, fatigue, gas, bloating, and a host of other symptoms and can also lead to poor nutrient absorption and intestinal disease.[6] This is why eating foods in proper combination, particularly avoiding starches and animal proteins in the same meal, can make digestion much more efficient and effective.

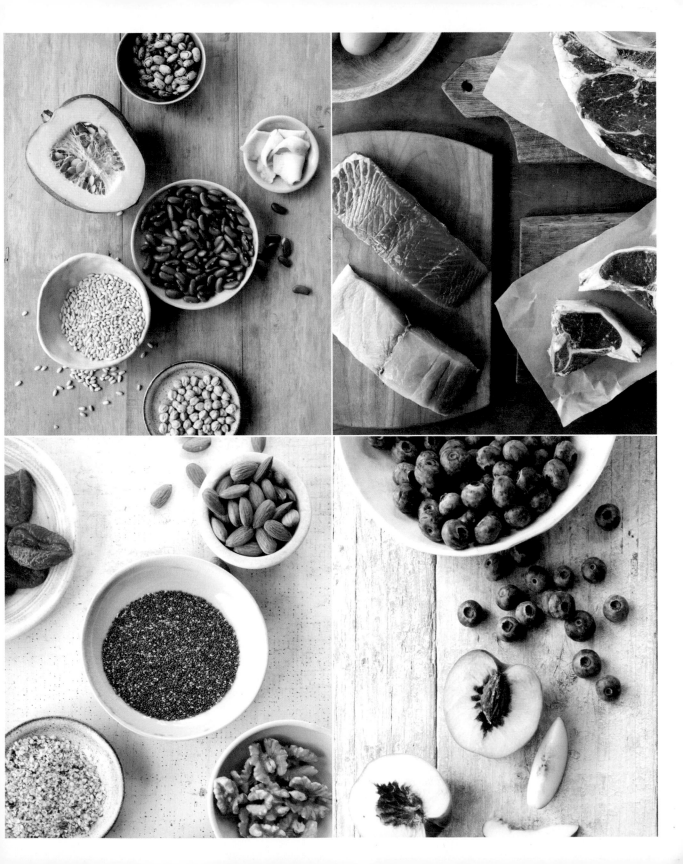

better digestion in three easy steps

STEP 1 *Pick just one category at each meal.*

FRESH FRUIT:

- Apples
- Bananas
- Oranges
- Pears
- Grapefruit
- Pineapple
- Melons
- Kiwi
- Grapes
- Berries
- Mango
- Papaya
- Peaches
- Nectarines
- Avocados

STARCHES:

- Butternut Squash
- Acorn Squash
- Kabocha Squash
- Sweet Potatoes
- Yams
- Avocados
- Young Thai Coconut Meat
- White Potatoes
- Wheat
- Barley
- Rye
- Oats
- Buckwheat
- Quinoa
- Amaranth
- Millet
- Spelt
- Pasta
- Cereals
- Cooked Corn
- Beans
- Lentils

ANIMAL PROTEIN:

- Red Meat
- Pork
- Poultry
- Fish
- Milk
- Cheese
- Yogurt
- Ice Cream
- Eggs

NUTS, SEEDS & DRIED FRUIT:

- Almonds
- Pecans
- Walnuts
- Brazil Nuts
- Macadamia Nuts
- Cashews
- Hazelnuts
- Sesame Seeds
- Sunflower Seeds
- Hemp Seeds
- Chia Seeds
- Flax Seeds
- Dried Fruit
- Mature Coconut
- Dried Coconut
- Bananas
- Avocados

STEP 2 Fill the rest of your plate with raw or cooked nonstarchy vegetables.

STEP 3 Wait 3 to 4 hours before switching categories.

If you become hungry between meals, feel free to snack on nonstarchy vegetables as much as desired.

NONSTARCHY VEGETABLES:

- Leafy Lettuces
- Cabbage
- Bok Choy
- Spinach
- Kale
- Broccoli
- Cauliflower
- Green Beans
- Spaghetti Squash
- Carrots
- Beets
- Onions
- Celery
- Cucumber
- Zucchini
- Yellow Summer Squash
- Raw Fresh Corn
- Fennel
- Artichokes
- Sprouts
- Scallions
- Bell Peppers
- Jalapeños
- Green Beans
- Sugar Snap Peas
- Asparagus
- Ginger
- Garlic
- Tomatoes

NEUTRAL ITEMS

that can also be enjoyed with any meal include:

- Butter
- Cold-Pressed Oils
- Lemons
- Limes
- Coconut Water
- Nondairy Nut or Seed Milks
- Heavy Cream
- Dark Chocolate (at least 70 percent cacao or higher)

EXCEPTIONS

There are a few exceptions to these basic rules:

- Fresh fruit is best eaten alone on an empty stomach, particularly melons, which are digested very quickly. Most fresh fruit can, however, be paired with raw leafy greens in salads or smoothies, without impeding digestion.

- Bananas can be combined with fresh fruits or with nuts, seeds, and dried fruit.

- Avocados can be combined with starches or with fresh fruit or with dried fruit.

- Beans and lentils are naturally more difficult to digest, but can be considered a starch for our purposes.

- Peanuts and soy nuts are not recommended due to their potential exposure to pesticides and mold.

NOTE: *I've generalized this approach to food combining to make the process easy and effective. While there are much more stringent guidelines out there, you don't have to overwhelm yourself with complicated rules until you've mastered these general concepts and want to simplify your meals even more. My approach will give you lasting results without compromising family dinners or your social schedule.*

This new way of eating may sound complicated at first, but it's actually quite simple once you get the hang of it. Craving a baked potato? Great! Enjoy that baked potato with a pat of real butter, a leafy green salad, and a side of roasted vegetables. Craving a steak? No problem. Enjoy it with a glass of wine, a juicy salad, and a pile of buttered vegetables. Craving pasta? Hold the cheese and smother it in rich marinara and your favorite veggies. Get the idea? You simply choose the one concentrated food you're craving most and create a healthy, vegetable-centric meal around that item. You're getting all of the flavors you love, while naturally balancing your plate.

It's this natural balancing act that makes these digestive principles so effective. Not only are you avoiding common junk food staples, like microwaved pizzas and double cheeseburgers, but you're also getting more nutritional bang for your buck. Studies have demonstrated that proteins and starches are not able to be digested fully when eaten together, which can lead to poor nutrient absorption.[7] When eaten separately, however, the body can assimilate your meal completely, allowing all of those vitamins and minerals to be properly absorbed. You'll feel so much better eating this way!

In fact, you may be wondering why this way of eating isn't more popular in our modern culture. The truth is, there is an unfortunate lack of peer-reviewed scientific research when it comes to food combining, which is why these digestive principles can be easily dismissed among modern health professionals. Though esteemed Paleo authors like Nora Gedgaudas and raw food pioneers like Ann Wigmore have all touted the benefits of eating foods in proper combinations, this approach remains relatively controversial and lacking in solid evidence at this time.

In light of this situation, I'd like to offer a few alternative explanations as to why these digestive principles are so effective when it comes to losing weight and improving overall health.

PROGRESS, NOT PERFECTION While I'm excited for you to take this leap, there's no need to dive in headfirst. This book is intended to make healthy eating easier and more enjoyable, and perfectionism is the fastest way to take all of the enjoyment out of eating. It's easy to get caught up in diet dogma, even with the simple goal of eating a "whole foods" diet, but keep in mind that our bodies are highly adaptable—they must be, since they seem to survive in spite of our junk food culture.

It bears repeating: you don't need to take drastic measures to see great results.

Rather than becoming militant about following food-combining rules and proclaiming all of your old favorite dishes off the table for good, aim to put these principles into practice and make healthier choices most of the time. Remember, a special holiday dinner, birthday party, or company barbecue is not going to make or break your new healthy habits. It's what you do the majority of the time that counts.

1. Food combining limits the variety of food and flavors on our plates. In other words, it makes our meals simpler. Studies have shown that humans have a tendency to overeat when we are offered a wide variety of foods during a meal.[8] So, by simplifying our meals, we will naturally eat less, without counting calories or worrying about portion sizes.

2. Food combining tends to reduce overall caloric intake. Even if you eat to your heart's content while following these digestive principles, it's likely that you'll be eating less, calorically speaking, because you'll be increasing your intake of nonstarchy vegetables. These vegetables are not only filling and low in calories, but they also provide a wide range of vitamins and minerals, which may help keep cravings at bay and the body functioning properly.

3 Food combining doesn't eliminate any (real) foods from your diet. This point is particularly important for those with a history of dieting. This method doesn't require giving up any of your favorite foods or eliminating entire food groups, which is critical for long-term enjoyment and success. When you enjoy what you're eating, you're more likely to stick with it! Plus, you'll avoid the dreaded cycle of restriction and bingeing that typically follows more stringent diet plans, along with the weight gain and guilt that come with it.

If nothing else, this approach encourages eating more fruits and vegetables and less processed and packaged foods, which is bound to have a positive impact on your health. If you're still skeptical of this new way of eating, there's no need to take my word for it. Try it for yourself and see how you feel. Your body comes equipped with all of the organs you need to detoxify, but they can do their job only when given the chance. Eating this way allows your body to function at its peak by reducing your digestive load and limiting toxic exposure. You may not even realize how good you can feel until you give it a shot.

YOUR EVERYDAY DETOX JUMP-START

Getting started with any new lifestyle change can be challenging, so I've included this jump-start to help you navigate the principles and recipes covered in this book. While you certainly don't need to follow any specific plan to enjoy these recipes, this section is for those of you looking for more guidance on how to put these digestive principles into practice on a regular basis. I can't wait for you to experience how easy this approach can be—eating delicious food while also enjoying improved digestion, better sleep, a clearer complexion, and increased energy while you reach your ideal weight.

This plan has been designed to be vegan-, vegetarian-, and omnivore-friendly, so it's highly adaptable to fit your needs. You can stick to the seven-day menu on page 14 or customize the program to your own preferences by using any other recipes found in this book. This meal plan adheres to all of the digestion principles discussed earlier, so the guesswork has already been done for you. Feel free to eat to your satisfaction, whether it's sticking to only liquid nourishment for breakfast or feasting like a king. I've included portion recommendations with each recipe, but these are only general guidelines—the portion size is ultimately up to you and your own unique appetite. Whatever you do, don't starve yourself. This lifestyle is not about restriction or deprivation—you can achieve your health goals while still eating hearty portions and even dessert.

EATING WELL YEAR-ROUND What is special about this everyday approach to detoxing is that there's no need to wait for the perfect time to cleanse. You won't need to isolate yourself from social situations or fear temptation, because eating this way won't disrupt your daily life. No matter what your schedule or excuse, you can always find a way to eat real food in real-life situations.

In many cases, short-term cleanses and detox programs are just another form of procrastination, allowing you to avoid the real task at hand—making lasting lifestyle change. Sure, juice fasts and cleanses may have their benefits, but it's far more important to learn how to feed yourself well on a regular basis. Instead of struggling with drastic measures for a week or two, why not start working on some easy, manageable habits right away? This could be as simple as starting each day with a healthy breakfast, or if you're feeling more ambitious, you can tackle several new habits at once. The choice is up to you! The more often you practice these new habits, the sooner they will become second nature, and before you know it, you'll automatically be making healthier choices on a daily basis.

TIPS TO PREPARE FOR THE WEEK AHEAD

If you can set aside just an hour of time to prepare a few key meal components for the week, like salad dressings and chopped vegetable toppings, you'll find that preparing homemade meals each weeknight can be surprisingly quick and easy.

By preparing ingredients like cauliflower and butternut squash "rice" ahead of time, you need to clean your food processor only once each week. If you have a shredding blade, you can quickly shred cabbage for coleslaw and a variety of vegetables for salad toppings, too. You'll be done with your food preparation for the entire week in less than an hour!

- Peel and freeze several ripe bananas to use for smoothies and ice cream. Depending on the power of your blender, you may want to slice the bananas into small coins before freezing to make blending easier.

- Peel, seed, and chop a butternut squash, then pulse it in a food processor to create "rice." (Store in the refrigerator to use for the Mexican Butternut Pilaf, page 119.)

- Pulse a head of cauliflower in a food processor to create "rice." (Store in the refrigerator to use for the Cauliflower Fried "Rice," page 120.)

- Wash and chop salad lettuce (or buy prewashed and chopped greens).

COOKING FOR ONE? Rather than making a different meal each night, simply prepare one or two family-size meals each week so you can enjoy easily reheated leftovers for the next several days. You can also prepare a large batch of salad toppings and a couple of homemade salad dressings for the week, which will make for convenient packed lunches.

- Wash and shred two heads of cabbage (or buy prewashed and shredded coleslaw mix).

- Wash and chop/shred any other salad toppings you may want for the week (such as chopped cucumber, bell peppers, tomatoes, beets, zucchini, carrots, and so on).

- Prepare a batch of Everyday Basil Vinaigrette (page 75) or Honey Dijon Dressing (page 73) to use for weeknight salads (these neutral dressings can be used interchangeably).

- Prepare a batch of Almond Butter Freezer Fudge (page 147) for the week.

- Prepare a large batch of Homemade Almond Milk (page 178; store in the refrigerator to use in smoothies and the Overnight Chia Pudding, page 59).

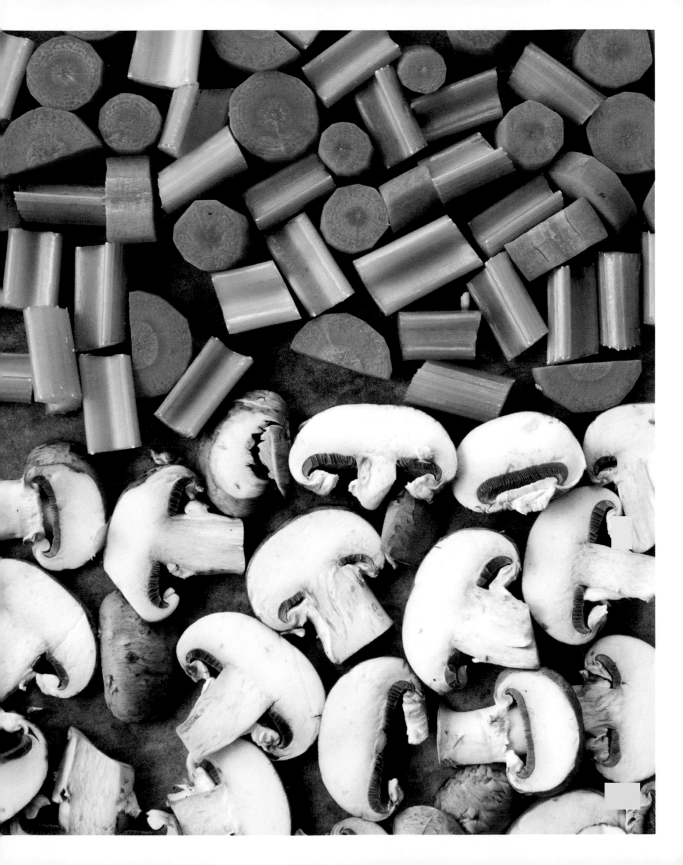

seven-day jump-start menu

The following menu exemplifies a week of detox-friendly meals, requiring minimal preparation.

NOTE: *Have a sweet tooth? You can enjoy a few pieces of dark chocolate (at least 70 percent cacao or higher) after any meal.*

MONDAY

Breakfast: Banana Nut Protein Shake (page 43)

Snack (optional): A ripe banana

Lunch: Chinese Cabbage Salad (page 80), topped with sliced avocado

Snack (optional): Dark Chocolate Pudding (page 146)

Dinner: Leafy green salad dressed with Everyday Basil Vinaigrette (page 75), followed by Cauliflower Fried "Rice" (page 120)

TUESDAY

Breakfast: Overnight Chia Pudding (page 59)

Snack (optional): A ripe banana

Lunch: Creamy Caesar Salad (page 81) with Walnut "Parmesan" (page 181)

Snack (optional): Almond Butter Freezer Fudge (page 147)

Dinner: Leafy green salad dressed with Everyday Basil Vinaigrette (page 75), followed by Mexican Butternut Pilaf (page 119) topped with sliced avocado

WEDNESDAY

Breakfast: Peachy Green Cleanser (page 51)

Snack (optional): Any piece of fruit

Lunch: Mediterranean Chopped Salad (page 84) topped with crumbled feta cheese

Snack (optional): Baby carrots or any other raw, nonstarchy veggies

Dinner: Leafy green salad dressed with Honey Dijon Dressing (page 73), followed by Maple Mustard Glazed Salmon (page 142) with Salt & Vinegar Brussels Sprouts (page 91)

THURSDAY

Breakfast: Kale Lemonade (page 38), followed by fresh fruit as desired

Snack (optional): Banana Coconut Muffin (page 56)

Lunch: Green salad topped with your favorite veggies and Hemp Seed Ranch (page 76)

Snack (optional): Baby carrots, or any other raw, nonstarchy veggies, dipped in extra Hemp Seed Ranch dressing

Dinner: Leafy green salad dressed with Honey Dijon Dressing (page 73), followed by a bowl of Broccoli Cheese Soup (page 101)

FRIDAY

Breakfast: Chocolate Chia Shake (page 48)

Snack (optional): Banana Coconut Muffin (page 56)

Lunch: No-Fail Kale Salad (page 83)

Snack (optional): Almond Butter Freezer Fudge (page 147)

Dinner: Leafy green salad dressed with Everyday Basil Vinaigrette (page 75), followed by Southwest Stuffed Sweet Potatoes (page 124)

SATURDAY

Breakfast: Maple Pecan Granola (page 54) with Homemade Almond Milk (page 178)

Snack (optional): A ripe banana

Lunch: Go-To Greek Salad (page 77)

Snack (optional): Sliced cucumber, or other raw, nonstarchy veggies

Dinner: Leafy green salad dressed with Everyday Basil Vinaigrette (page 75), followed by Pantry Pad Thai (page 137)

SUNDAY

Breakfast: Caramelized Onion & Red Bell Pepper Frittata (page 65) with a mixed green salad

Snack (optional): Handful of cherry tomatoes

Lunch: Raw Falafel Wraps (page 106)

Snack (optional): Crispy Zucchini Chips (page 95)

Dinner: Roasted Vegetable Salad with Shallot Vinaigrette (page 78)

SHOPPING LIST FOR THE SEVEN-DAY MEAL PLAN

To make this jump-start incredibly easy for you to try, below I've provided a list of the ingredients you'll need for the entire week. The quantities assume that you are going to feed two to four people. If you're feeding only yourself, buy half of the fresh ingredients listed or feel free to make family-size portions and freeze the extras for easy meals in the future.

Fresh Produce:

2 dozen bananas
2 Fuji apples
1 pound baby spinach
2 pounds mixed salad greens
5 heads romaine lettuce
2 bunches curly kale
1 bunch Lacinato (Dino) kale
1 bunch collard leaves
2 heads cabbage or 3 (12-ounce) bags shredded cabbage
1 pound brussels sprouts
5 avocados
1 (2½-pound) head cauliflower or 1 (2-pound) bag cauliflower florets
1 (2½-pound) butternut squash
1 (3½-pound) spaghetti squash
2 pounds fresh broccoli
4 sweet potatoes
4 pounds fresh tomatoes
3 Roma tomatoes

2 pounds carrots
4 cucumbers
1 large zucchini
7 red bell peppers
3 red onions
3 yellow onions
1 pound asparagus
2 jalapeños
2 pounds lemons
1 lime
1 bunch celery
1 bunch fresh cilantro
1 bunch fresh parsley
1 bunch fresh dill
1 bunch fresh basil
1 bunch green onions
Fresh ginger
Fresh garlic bulb
Shallot
Medjool dates
Olives
Mung bean sprouts (optional)
Fresh fruit, as desired (optional)
1 pint cherry tomatoes (optional)
Baby carrots (optional)

Animal Protein:

1½ dozen eggs
1 pound wild salmon
4 ounces chèvre (soft goat cheese)
2 (6-ounce) blocks raw goat feta

Freezer Section:

1 (10-ounce) bag frozen peaches
1 (10-ounce) bag frozen pineapple
1 (12-ounce) bag frozen artichoke hearts

Pantry Staples:

Raw apple cider vinegar
Coconut vinegar
Extra-virgin olive oil
Coconut oil
Grass-fed butter (optional)
Coconut flour
Shredded unsweetened coconut
Honey (raw, clover, or both)
Dijon mustard
Tamari or coconut aminos
Sriracha sauce

Nutritional yeast
Toasted sesame oil
Raw cacao powder or cocoa powder
Maple syrup (preferably Grade B)
Vanilla extract
Ground cinnamon
Ground nutmeg
Ground cumin
Ground coriander
Chili powder
Dried oregano
Dried chives
Dried parsley
Dried dill
Onion powder
Baking soda
Sea salt
Black pepper

Nuts, Seeds & Dried Fruit:

Almond butter
Hemp hearts
Hulled sunflower seeds
Pecans
Walnuts
Cashews
Almonds, whole and slivered
Golden raisins
Chia seeds

MAXIMIZE YOUR RESULTS

The following tips will help you get the most out of this book, whether you're looking to lose weight, strengthen your digestion, or simply feel more energetic throughout your day. Making a few minor changes to your daily routine can add up to big results, so feel free to try one, or all, of these ideas to ensure you reach your goals.

Properly combine your meals.

If you do nothing else, adhering to the digestion principles discussed earlier in the chapter will naturally balance your day by encouraging you to make mindful choices at each and every meal. Remember, you can still enjoy the foods you love—just not necessarily all at the same time. All of the recipes in this book are labeled by food category (such as animal protein, starch, or nut/seed/dried fruit) to make these principles even easier to follow. Be sure to wait three to four hours between your meals before switching categories, and feel free to snack on neutral foods, like nonstarchy vegetables, at any time of the day.

Begin each meal with something raw.

Raw plant foods are hydrating, filling, and bursting with nutrition. The more often you eat them, the more inclined you may be to keep eating well for the rest of the day! Before you dig into your main course, make a habit of snacking on a handful of raw vegetables before lunch and enjoying a leafy green salad before dinner each evening. Not only will these veggies prepare your palate for a healthy meal, but you'll also benefit from their raw enzymes, which may boost digestion. Of course, you can always enjoy a large salad, with filling toppings, as your main course, too.

Limit caffeine and alcohol intake.

Coffee, tea, alcohol, and soda are all dehydrating and acidic in the body and may inhibit nutrient absorption and stress the adrenal glands. You can still enjoy your favorite morning beverage in moderation, but avoid drinking caffeinated beverages with, or immediately after, your meals for best digestion and nutrient absorption. If you choose to consume alcohol, stick to just the occasional glass of wine with dinner.

Limit animal protein.

Aim to eat no more than 25 grams of protein per meal, as the body will struggle to process and assimilate more than this amount in one sitting.[9] For reference, this amount of protein can be found in a 3-ounce serving of meat or fish, which is about the size of a deck of cards. This portion may be significantly smaller than what you have come to expect from a restaurant, but keep in mind that excess protein is converted into sugar and may be stored as fat in the body. Instead of overdosing on protein, fill up the rest of your plate with fiber-rich veggies to keep your overall meal balanced and satisfying.

WHERE DO YOU GET YOUR PROTEIN? The beauty of this lifestyle is that there's no need to give up meat if you don't want to—it's perfect for vegetarians and meat-eaters alike. While meat, fish, and eggs are generally considered to be complete sources of protein, keep in mind that the protein they contain can't be assimilated by the body until it is broken down into amino acids first. Amino acids, also known as the building blocks of protein, are used to create the type of protein that the human body can actually utilize, and they happen to be found in a variety of fruits, vegetables, nuts, and seeds as well. In fact, up to 50 percent of the calories found in green vegetables can come from protein,[10] so there is very little risk of becoming protein-deficient as long as you consume a varied diet loaded with whole foods.

Limit sugar consumption.

Studies show that consumption of refined sugar can harm metabolism, speed up the aging process, and may contribute to the prevalence of obesity and diabetes.[11] Our bodies are designed to crave sweets, preferably in the form of naturally sweet fruits, which are bursting with vitamins, minerals, and antioxidants. But unfortunately, we can also find ourselves craving sweets that aren't as beneficial to us, such as sodas, candy bars, and baked goods. The more often we give in to the urge for these refined-sugar treats, the more often we will crave them, perpetuating an endless cycle of sugar cravings and energy crashes. As you adjust to this lifestyle, you may find it helpful to limit your sugar consumption for a week or two in order to reacclimate your taste buds and squash your refined-sugar cravings for good. To make the transition easier, enjoy a fruit-based smoothie (see chapter 3) or a bowl of Banana Soft Serve (page 162) for a naturally sweetened treat.

MAKING THIS PROGRAM WORK FOR YOU

What I love about this approach to detoxing is that it can work for anyone, in any situation. When I started adhering to these digestive principles myself, one of my top priorities at mealtime was saving room for dessert. I loved that I could plan each one of my meals around my sweet tooth—enjoying a treat after both lunch and dinner daily! For example, if I wanted a raw nut-based dessert, like a Peppermint Fudge Bar (page 166) after my meal, I'd enjoy a large salad first, dressed with Creamy Jalapeño Dressing (page 72), so that it would be easily digested with my treat. If sweets aren't your thing, but you crave a good steak, a buttered potato, or a favorite glass of wine, you can always base your meal choices around one of these items instead. Practically any favorite can fit into this detox lifestyle, so you'll never have to feel deprived while working toward your health goals.

Now, let's get started!

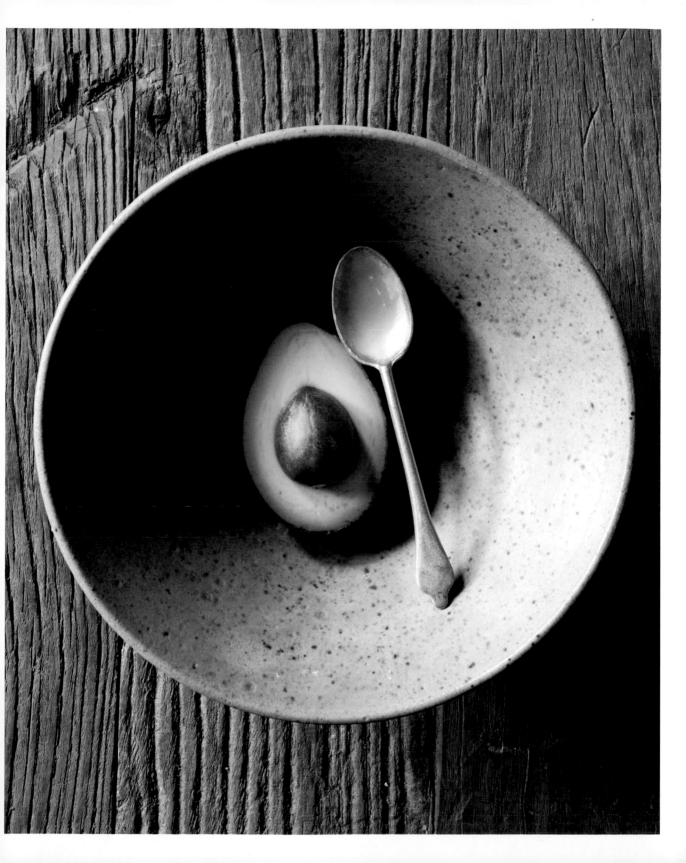

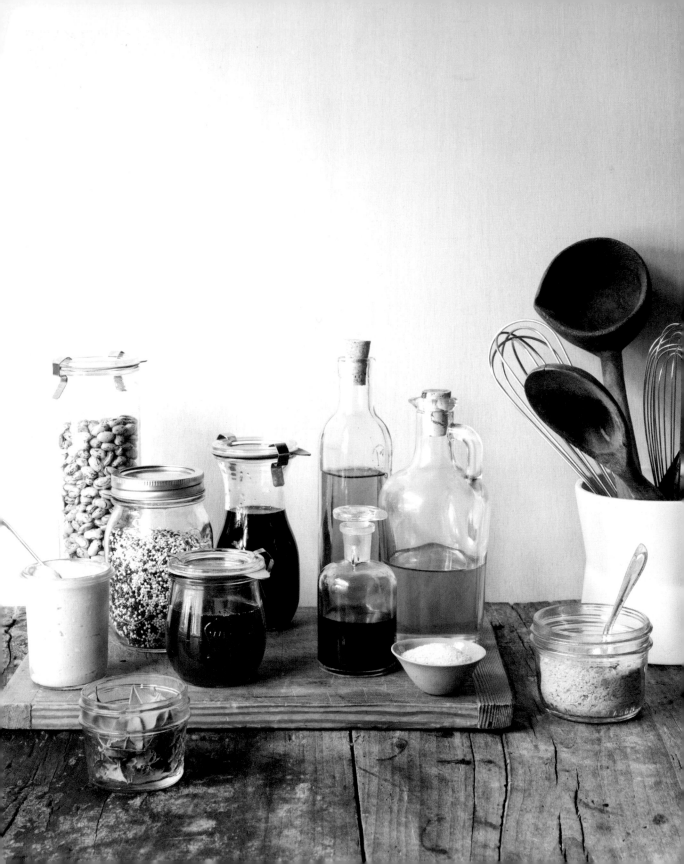

stocking your detox-friendly kitchen

CHAPTER 2

Before we get to the recipes, let's take a look at your kitchen. Do you have easy access to a blender? What types of foods and ingredients do you stock in your refrigerator and pantry? It's likely that you'll use and consume whatever is handy, so one of the best ways to set yourself up for success is to have detox-friendly tools and ingredients easily accessible. By simply upgrading the items in your pantry, you'll automatically make better choices daily.

PANTRY ESSENTIALS

The following staples are key to creating mouth-watering dishes without compromising your health. They can easily be found at your local Whole Foods Market, natural health food store, or through various online retailers. For easy online shopping, visit www.detoxinista.com/resources.

Almond Flour (Blanched) & Almond Meal

A grain-free alternative to wheat flour, blanched almond flour is made by simply grinding blanched almonds into a fine powder. Similarly, almond meal is made by grinding whole almonds with their skins intact, resulting in a coarser grind. If you don't mind your baked goods speckled with ground almond skins and a slightly more cakelike texture, then almond meal is a more economical option when compared to using blanched almond flour and is the ingredient I prefer to use most often. Keep in mind that almonds have the potential to oxidize and create acrylamide, a harmful carcinogen, when baked at high heat, so these nut-based flours should be used only in moderation and baked at low temperatures.

CUT YOUR CANCER RISK Acrylamide is a carcinogen that has been found to cause cancer in laboratory animals. This chemical is not added to food but is created naturally when certain foods are roasted, fried, or baked, particularly French fries, potato chips, coffee, almonds, crackers, and bread. It is nearly impossible to avoid this chemical altogether, as it occurs naturally in a wide range of plant foods and animal products, but you can limit your exposure by using safer cooking methods, such as steaming and boiling, cooking susceptible foods at lower temperatures, and avoiding meats, vegetables, and starches that are darkly browned or charred. You'll notice that all of the recipes in this book that call for heating raw nuts are kept to temperatures of 250°F or lower, to avoid browning and reduce the potential formation of acrylamide.

Apple Cider Vinegar (Raw)

This naturally fermented vinegar is rich in minerals, like potassium and calcium, and is easy to recognize by the cloudy debris floating in the bottle, called "the mother." Though it may not look very appealing, this strandlike debris is a sign that the vinegar contains live enzymes and bacteria that may promote better digestion. Select a bottle that is organic and labeled "with the mother" for best quality.

Buckwheat Flour

Contrary to its name, buckwheat is actually a seed and has absolutely no relation to wheat. You can create this gluten-free flour at home by grinding raw buckwheat groats in a blender or coffee grinder, resulting in a light-colored and mild-flavored baking ingredient. It can also be purchased at your local natural grocer, but the store-bought version will be darker in color and more bitter in flavor, because the darker hulls are included when ground. Buck-wheat has a very distinct and strong flavor, so it is not recommended as a substitute for traditional flour.

Butter (Grass-Fed)

Skip the butter substitutes and enjoy the real thing. Grass-fed butter is a great source of vitamins A, D, E, K, and K2 and aids in the absorption of fat-soluble vitamins. This butter is particularly nutrient-rich because it's made from the milk of cows that were allowed to graze on grass, rather than those that are confined to eating soy- and corn-based feeds. Popular grass-fed brands include Kerrygold and Organic Valley (sold as pasture butter), but if you have difficulty locating them in your area, simply look for organic butter when possible, to avoid added antibiotics and hormones. Like coconut oil, real butter also remains stable at high heat, making it an ideal option for cooking.

Cacao Powder (Raw) and Cocoa Powder

Cacao is the raw ingredient used to make chocolate and is rich in antioxidants, magnesium, and iron.

I recommend using raw cacao powder when adding a chocolate flavor to a smoothie or no-bake dessert and saving the cocoa powder in your pantry for working with oven-baked goods. Flavorwise, raw cacao and cocoa powder can be used interchangeably with very little difference in taste, but the raw cacao will provide a significantly higher antioxidant boost compared to Dutch-processed cocoa.

Chocolate Chips (Dark)

Aim to buy dark chocolate chips (70 percent cacao or higher) to avoid too many unnecessary additives. Brands are available that are vegan, dairy-free, soy-free, and even sugar-free, to meet any other special dietary needs you may have.

Coconut (Shredded Unsweetened)

Not to be confused with the moist and sweetened coconut that is often called for in traditional baking recipes, shredded unsweetened coconut has been dehydrated, so it's drier in texture and has only one ingredient on the label—coconut.

Coconut Aminos

A soy-free and gluten-free alternative to soy sauce, this liquid condiment adds a salty flavor to any dish and has a higher amino acid content than regular soy sauce. Keep in mind that coconut aminos contain less sodium than tamari or soy sauce, so you may want to increase the amount used, or add an extra pinch of salt, when making recipe substitutions.

Coconut Flour

This flour is uniquely absorbent and makes an excellent baking alternative for those who must remain gluten-free or grain-free. Because it is so absorbent, coconut flour also tends to be a more economical option when compared to other grain-free flours—a little goes a long way! Be sure to use coconut flour only in recipes that have been specifically developed for this special flour, as it cannot be substituted for any other flour. When measuring coconut flour, use the "scoop and sweep" method for

DON'T FEAR SATURATED FAT Saturated fat was once vilified as a contributor to high cholesterol and heart disease, but a study in *The American Journal of Clinical Nutrition* found that saturated fat intake is not associated with an increased risk of coronary heart disease, stroke, or cardiovascular disease.[1] On the contrary, much of the saturated fat found in coconut oil is lauric acid, a medium-chain fatty acid that contains antibacterial, antimicrobial, and antiviral properties, which are thought to support the immune system.

You might be surprised to hear that eating foods rich in saturated fat, like pure coconut oil and grass-fed butter, may actually promote weight loss, too. Back in the 1940s, farmers fed their livestock coconut oil in an attempt to fatten them up, but much to their dismay, the animals became leaner as a result! Recent studies have shown that coconut oil can promote a reduction in abdominal fat in human subjects, as well.[2] As an added bonus, cooking with grass-fed butter and coconut oil helps the body absorb the fat-soluble vitamins naturally found in certain vegetables.

accurate results: simply scoop the measuring cup into the container of coconut flour, then sweep the top with the back of a knife to remove the excess. Even just an extra teaspoon of coconut flour can affect the texture of a recipe, so be sure to measure carefully.

Coconut Oil

The most appealing aspect of coconut oil is its stability—it can be stored for long periods of time without becoming rancid, and it is safe for cooking at high heat. It's also uniquely solid at temperatures below 76°F, making it the perfect thickener for raw and no-bake recipes. Refined coconut oil can be used at higher cooking temperatures and provides a more neutral flavor, but I prefer to use cold-pressed, extra-virgin coconut oil in all of my recipes, as it is the least processed version available.

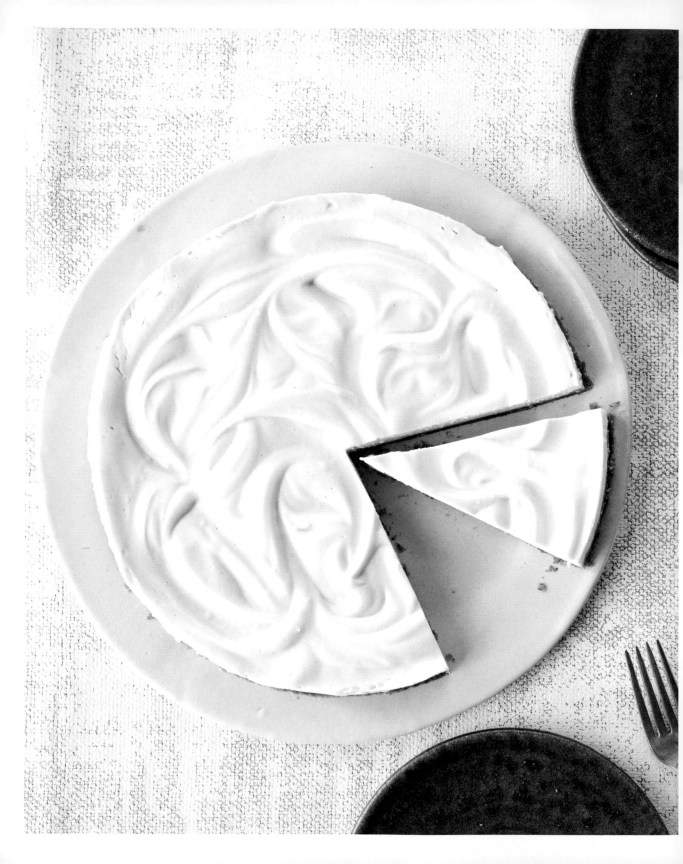

Coconut Vinegar (Raw)

This vinegar is relatively new to the market, but it's becoming quite popular due to its superior nutritional profile. Raw coconut vinegar contains a number of amino acids, broad-spectrum B vitamins, vitamin C, and a naturally occurring prebiotic to promote digestion, making it an excellent addition to your favorite salad dressing. Make sure you select a brand that is organic and unpasteurized to maximize the potential health benefits.

Dairy Products

Milk has been marketed as a healthy beverage for years, but there is little evidence to support the idea that dairy consumption promotes bone health or prevents osteoporosis. In fact, a twelve-year Harvard study of nearly seventy-eight thousand women demonstrated that higher milk consumption led to a significantly higher risk of hip and bone fracture.[3]

However, this doesn't mean that dairy can't be enjoyed as part of a healthy diet. You can use dairy as a tool to make vegetables taste better, which may in turn lead to an overall increase in your vegetable consumption. Dairy products made from goat or sheep's milk, particularly those that are raw and unpasteurized, are considered easier to digest than those made from pasteurized cow's milk (see the sidebar above right), so they are a tasty alternative to traditional favorites. Several of the recipes in this book call for raw goat Cheddar, Pecorino Romano (made from sheep's milk), or pasteurized goat's milk yogurt, all of which are available at Whole Foods Markets across the country, as well as at local health food stores. My favorite brands include Alta Dena, Capretta, Mt. Sterling, and Redwood Hill Farm.

NOTE: *The U.S. Food and Drug Administration (FDA) requires that cheese made from raw, unpasteurized milk must be aged for sixty days to be considered safe for public sale in grocery stores. This aging process allows the acids and salt found in cheese to naturally destroy harmful bacteria without the use of heat.*

WHY IS GOAT'S MILK BETTER? Goat's milk is often thought of as a hypoallergenic alternative to cow's milk, as its protein structure is significantly different, containing less of the allergenic alpha S1 casein protein. Goat's milk has been studied as a substitute for cow's milk in children, and over a five-month period, those receiving goat's milk excelled in weight gain, height, and nutrition, when compared to children on cow's milk. In studies of children with allergies to cow's milk, treatment with goat's milk produced positive results in 93 percent of subjects, which also suggests that goat's milk is easier to digest and less allergenic.[4] Since goat and sheep's milks are structurally similar, feel free to enjoy them both as an alternative to cow dairy.

Dates

Also known as "nature's candy," this fiber-rich fruit is incredibly sweet and happens to be a great source of several vitamins and minerals. Loaded with calcium, iron, potassium, copper, and magnesium, dates have been associated with relief from constipation, intestinal disorders, heart problems, anemia, abdominal cancer, and many other conditions. Medjool dates are the variety I prefer to use in recipes, as they are commonly found in most grocery stores.

Dijon Mustard

This richly flavored mustard adds a delicious acidity to certain recipes, but be sure to look for brands with no added sugar in the ingredients.

Eggs (Pasture-Raised)

When buying eggs, look for organic and pasture-raised varieties for the greatest nutrition content. Studies have shown that, when compared to conventional eggs, eggs from pastured hens may contain roughly half the cholesterol, 50 percent more vitamin E, and three times more beta-carotene.[5] If pasture-raised eggs aren't in the budget, be sure to look for organic varieties in order to avoid the arsenic and antibiotics that are often fed to factory-farmed chicken.

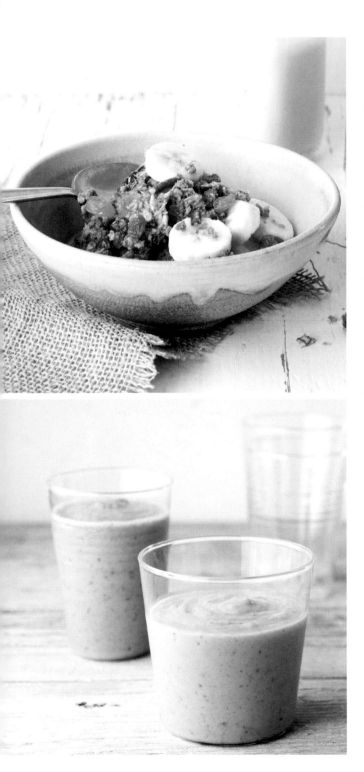

Extra-Virgin Olive Oil

This cold-pressed oil has been recognized for its anti-inflammatory benefits, making it an excellent addition to salad dressings. Studies have associated the monounsaturated fatty acids found in olive oil with a decreased risk of cardiovascular disease, a decrease in blood pressure, and improved blood sugar regulation.[6] However, because this delicate oil can be damaged when cooking at temperatures near 300°F, it's not recommended for use in high-heat cooking. (Stick to heat-stable butter or coconut oil instead.)

Fruit (Dried)

When selecting dried fruit, be sure to look for varieties that are free of added sulfites or sugars. Since these fruits are highly concentrated, it's also a good idea to buy organic varieties, to avoid consuming a concentrated dose of the contaminants found on conventionally grown fruit.

Hemp Hearts

The most nutritious part of the hemp seed, hemp hearts are the tender inner kernels that can be eaten straight from the package. They are loaded with easily digested plant-based protein, containing all of the essential amino acids, and they provide an ideal ratio of omega-6 to omega-3 fatty acids, which can help prevent inflammation in the body. They're perfect for making nut-free and dairy-free milk (see page 176) and add an extra dose of protein to any smoothie.

Herbs and Spices (Dried)

Dried herbs and spices are convenient and economical alternatives to the fresh varieties, thanks to their concentrated flavors and long shelf life. Since these dried plants are so concentrated, be sure to select organic varieties whenever possible, to avoid a potentially concentrated dose of pesticides. When substituting dried herbs for fresh in a recipe, just one-third of the amount is required (for example, 1 teaspoon dried herbs = 1 tablespoon fresh herbs).

Honey (Raw)

This type of honey has not been heated or pasteurized, allowing it to maintain all of its naturally occurring vitamins, enzymes, and antioxidants. Raw honey is not only known for its antiviral, antibacterial, and antifungal properties, but it may also help strengthen the immune system and reduce allergies. I prefer to use raw honey in recipes that won't be heated, in order to retain its naturally occurring nutrients, but for all other recipes, regular honey (such as clover honey) can be used as a more economical option, particularly in baked desserts.

Maple Syrup

Made from maple tree sap, this natural sweetener offers a rich, almost caramel-like sweetness that is an excellent source of manganese and a good source of zinc, both of which are essential for a healthy immune system. Be sure to select a bottle that is 100 percent pure maple syrup, without any other ingredients or fillers. For a more robust maple flavor and higher mineral content, I use Grade B maple syrup in all of my recipes.

Meat

Though all of the recipes in this book are meat-free, I've noted when the addition of high-quality meat would be appropriate for my omnivore readers. Look for grass-fed and pasture-raised meats when possible, as these animals not only are more ethically raised, but also tend to be more nutritious. Additionally, choosing organically raised cuts will help you avoid the added hormones and antibiotics given to conventionally raised animals. Consuming charred meat may increase the risk of certain cancers,[7] so stick to gently stewed or baked meat as often as possible.

A NOTE ON ZERO-CALORIE SWEETENERS

Though they have become popular for managing sugar and calorie intake, artificial sweeteners may disrupt the hormonal and neurological signals in the body that control hunger. A study of rats that were fed artificially sweetened food found that their metabolism slowed down and they were triggered to consume more calories and gain more weight than rats fed sugar-sweetened food.[8] This is why the recipes included in this book call for all-natural sweeteners, which are more likely to help keep your hormones and appetite properly balanced.

For those who must avoid even the natural sweeteners, the South American herb stevia may be a safe all-natural sugar alternative. Keep in mind, however, that its sweet taste could still trick the body into thinking it's actually receiving sugar, which may lead to a negative impact on blood sugar and hunger regulation in certain individuals. If you do choose to use stevia, be sure to buy a pure brand without many additives or extra ingredients and use it in moderation.

Nutritional Yeast

This deactivated yeast is often sold as yellow flakes and provides a nutty, "cheesy" flavor to a variety of dairy-free dishes. Nutritional yeast is a complete protein, containing all nine essential amino acids, and is typically considered safe for those on a yeast-cleansing program.

Nuts and Seeds (Raw)

When eaten in moderation, nuts have been associated with a variety of benefits, including decreased body mass index and lower blood pressure. Be sure to select nuts and seeds that are raw and organic whenever possible, as roasting their delicate oils can lead to oxidation and the formation of acrylamide, a harmful carcinogen. (See "Cut Your Cancer Risk," page 22.) For best digestion, soak nuts and seeds in pure water before consuming them (see the soaking chart below).

PLEASE NOTE: *As of September 1, 2007, almonds that are grown in the United States must be pasteurized before they are sold. These almonds may be steam-heated or exposed to propylene oxide gas to meet these requirements (fumigation with propylene oxide is not allowed if the almonds will be sold as certified organic) and can still be labeled as "raw" for sale. If you'd prefer to purchase truly raw almonds, you can still buy them directly from an almond grower at a local farmers' market or look for imported Italian raw almonds at most health food stores or online.*

Produce (Fresh)

Select organic fruits and vegetables as often as your budget and resources allow to limit your exposure to pesticide residues. If buying all organic produce isn't feasible, be sure to check out the Dirty Dozen list produced by the Environmental Working Group (www.ewg.org) each year. This list reports the fruits

SOAKING FOR BETTER DIGESTION If you find nuts and seeds particularly difficult to digest, soaking them may help. Nuts and seeds naturally contain enzyme inhibitors and phytic acid, which can prevent mineral absorption and cause digestive discomfort, but exposing them to moisture can help reduce or remove these substances by mimicking the germination process. Soaking times vary depending on the type of nut or seed used, but the overall process is the same. Simply cover the nuts or seeds in pure water to soak for the appropriate amount of time, then discard the soaking water and rinse well. Soaked nuts can be briefly stored in the fridge, but for best shelf life, dry them thoroughly. You can use a dehydrator to dry them for up to twenty-four hours, or use an oven at the lowest setting—at a temperature no higher than 150°F—to keep the enzymes and delicate oils intact. Soaked nuts and seeds will plump and expand, so be sure to use a container that will accommodate the nuts or seeds swelling two to three times in volume. The recipes in this book typically call for dry nuts and seeds, so unless noted otherwise, make sure your ingredients are not wet for best results.

Recommended soaking times for common nuts and seeds:

- **Almonds:** 8 hours
- **Brazil nuts:** 3 hours
- **Cashews:** 2 hours
- **Hazelnuts:** 8 hours
- **Macadamia nuts:** 8 hours
- **Pecans:** 6 hours
- **Pine nuts:** 6 hours
- **Pumpkin seeds, hulled:** 6 hours
- **Sesame seeds:** 8 hours
- **Sunflower seeds, hulled:** 2 hours
- **Walnuts:** 4 hours

Don't have the time or energy to soak your nuts or seeds? Don't sweat it. Remember, we aren't aiming for perfection here, and keeping things as easy as possible is key to creating lasting lifestyle change. By simply upgrading the quality of the foods you consume on a regular basis, you'll be making great strides in your health and digestion, so there's no need to complicate things if this process sounds overwhelming. Unsoaked nuts and seeds should not have a huge impact on your digestion when eaten in moderation, and they are still a much better choice over any processed snack.

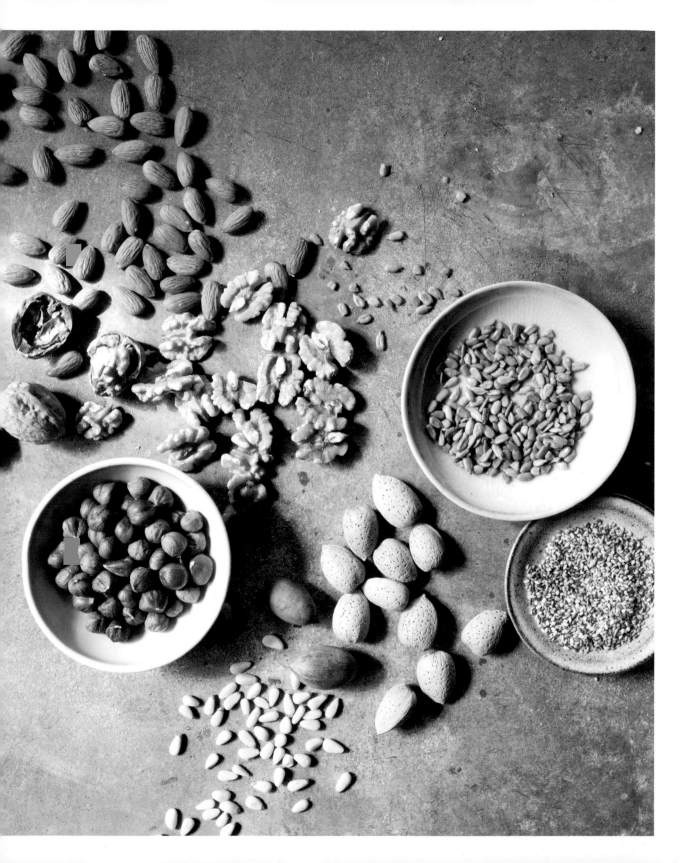

and vegetables that are most exposed to pesticides, so you can make an informed choice when shopping. Regardless, eating any fruits and vegetables is still better than eating none at all!

Quinoa (pronounced KEEN-wah)

This pseudograin cooks similar to a grain but is actually a gluten-free seed. Quinoa is a complete protein, containing all nine essential amino acids, and is a good source of fiber and phosphorous, along with magnesium and iron. For a nutrient-rich alternative, try using quinoa instead of rice in your favorite stir-fries and curries.

Sea Salt

I use pink Himalayan or Celtic sea salt in all of my recipes, as they are unrefined and unbleached and contain a full spectrum of minerals and trace elements, including iodine. The key to shopping for salt is to take note of its color—full-spectrum salt will always have a pink or sandy, nonwhite color, while white salts have typically been stripped of their mineral content. I prefer to use finely ground sea salt in all of my recipes for an evenly distributed flavor.

Seafood

Fish is an easily digested source of protein that is loaded with omega-3 fatty acids, which may prevent inflammation and promote healthy heart and brain function. Due to potential contamination, stick to smaller varieties of fish, which tend to be less polluted than larger ones, and look for wild-caught options as often as possible. Additionally, the FDA recommends that children and pregnant women should consume no more than 12 ounces of low-mercury fish per week. Stay up-to-date on the safest varieties of fish in your area by visiting www.seafoodwatch.org.

Tamari

A gluten-free soy sauce, tamari has a smoother and richer taste than regular soy sauce and is easily found in most grocery stores. Tamari makes a great

WHY GLUTEN-FREE? Gluten is a type of protein that occurs naturally in several types of grains, including wheat, spelt, barley, and rye, and in our modern culture, intolerance and sensitivity to this gluelike protein is on the rise. For individuals with celiac disease, an autoimmune disorder, the body recognizes gluten as a foreign invader to the body, causing the immune system to attack not only the gluten, but also the intestinal wall itself, leading to nutrient deficiencies and a host of other health issues. To make matters worse, studies have shown that more than 80 percent of people with celiac disease don't even know they have it.[9] One study has shown that gluten can cause gastrointestinal symptoms even in subjects without celiac disease, including pain, bloating, and fatigue, without their immune system producing antibodies (which is how gluten intolerance is currently measured).[10] Simply put, you don't have to have celiac disease or gluten sensitivity to have a reaction to gluten.

To accommodate the increasing numbers of people who are finding themselves sensitive to gluten, all of the recipes in this book have been developed using grain-free alternatives, like coconut flour and almond meal, as well as gluten-free pseudograins, like buckwheat and quinoa. Nutritionally, you won't miss any vitamins or minerals by eliminating wheat and other grains, since those same nutrients can all be easily found in other food sources, especially when consuming a diet rich in fruits, vegetables, nuts, and seeds. Just like the digestion principles discussed earlier, you may not know how good you can feel without gluten unless you give it a try.

salt substitute in a variety of recipes, but be sure to check the label to ensure that the soy products you select are free of MSG and certified organic, to avoid genetically modified ingredients. If gluten-free recipes are not a priority for you, soy sauce can be used as a substitute in most cases.

HELPFUL KITCHEN TOOLS

You don't need much more than a cutting board and a good knife to create an array of healthy dishes, but the following tools can make life a little easier. While there's no need to buy them all, and certainly not all at once, as you start enjoying these vegetable-centric meals more often, you may find yourself collecting quite a few of these kitchen appliances to save on prep time.

Bakeware

Choose baking pans without a nonstick coating. The best options include stoneware, glass, stainless steel, ceramic, and enameled cast iron. If you can't replace your nonstick bakeware, be sure to never place it in an oven hotter than 500°F and use a liner to prevent food from coming into direct contact with its surface. I like to use rimmed baking sheets when working with chopped vegetables so I don't have to worry about them falling off the edge when moving the sheets in and out of the oven.

Box Grater

This handy tool is perfect for shredding hard cheeses by hand, and it can also be used to grate raw cauliflower florets, creating a quick ricelike texture without the need for a food processor.

Coffee Grinder

This small machine offers an affordable way to grind small batches of nuts, seeds, and grains into fine homemade flour.

Cutting Board

Any type of cutting board will do, but wood and bamboo cutting boards are best for keeping your knives sharp. If you work with raw meat, you may want to invest in a separate board for vegetables to prevent cross-contamination.

Food Processor

A food processor is similar to a blender, but it's handy for large jobs that require some texture, like when you want to gently process vegetables into a ricelike consistency. It can also quickly slice or shred veggies and create homemade nut butters. I recommend selecting a large-capacity food processor for making family-size batches of vegetable "rice," shredded salad toppings, and blended soups.

Glass Mason Jars

Glass jars are my favorite way to store salad dressings and leftovers, as these affordable and reusable containers won't leach toxic chemicals into your food. Many items, like nut butters and jelly, come in glass jars with screw-on lids already, so you could easily have a steady supply of storage containers for life.

Good Knife

A sharp knife is key to kitchen safety when slicing and chopping vegetables. A dull knife may slip while trying to slice through a juicy tomato, but a sharp one will cut exactly where you intend it to cut. I personally love ceramic knives, as they stay sharp forever, but you may also want to invest in a sturdy metal chef's knife for cutting into the tough shells of winter squash.

High-Speed Blender

If you plan on preparing dairy-free sauces and leafy green smoothies on a regular basis, this tool is a worthy investment. It can pulverize anything and everything into a smooth and creamy consistency in just a matter of seconds, saving you quite a bit of time and effort. A conventional blender will also do the trick in most cases, but keep in mind that the results may not turn out as smooth and creamy as intended.

Immersion Blender

This stick blender can be used directly in a cooking pot to blend hot soups, eliminating the need to transfer batches to a food processor or blender. Though the texture won't be quite as smooth as when using a traditional blender, the convenience is hard to beat.

Juicer

If you're interested in embarking on a regular juicing regimen, investing in a juicer is an economical choice when compared to buying individual juices from a juice bar. Unlike a blender, a juicer grinds fruits and vegetables and then separates the pulp from the juice, leaving you with pure liquid nourishment. The two most common types of juicers on the market are centrifugal and masticating. Centrifugal juicers are often seen at fresh juice bars, and this is the type of juicer I recommend for beginners, as it is the cheapest and fastest option. Masticating juicers are typically more expensive and slower, but they produce a higher-quality juice by gently "chewing" the produce, which reduces the oxidation of the resulting juice and allows you to store it for up to 48 hours in the refrigerator.

Kitchen Scale

When working with fresh produce, a kitchen scale comes in handy for accurately measuring pounds and ounces.

Mandoline Slicer

This tool is handy for creating ultrathin, uniform slices. Use it to make zucchini "noodles" for my Zucchini Lasagna (page 139) or to slice paper-thin vegetables for homemade baked chips (see page 95).

Microplane Grater

This ultrafine grater is perfect for quickly adding fresh spices to a dish, like garlic, ginger, or nutmeg. I often use a Microplane to add raw garlic to a recipe instead of using a knife to mince, because it's faster and provides a more uniform flavor throughout.

Mini Food Chopper

If you're not quite ready to invest in a food processor, or you'd simply like an easier option for smaller jobs, a mini food chopper (also called a mini food processor) can be useful. I still use the same one I've owned since college, and it's perfect for whipping up a batch of hummus, pudding, or individual batches of cauliflower "rice."

Nontoxic Cookware

Choose pans without a synthetic nonstick coating, which may leach chemicals into your food and environment when heated. My favorite options include cast-iron, ceramic, and stainless steel cookware. Traditional cast iron is very affordable and becomes naturally nonstick with frequent use and proper seasoning. Alternatively, you can choose enameled cast iron, which doesn't require any seasoning to create a nonstick quality and is often dishwasher-safe. When working with ceramic-coated and stainless steel cookware, be sure to use non-abrasive cleaners to prevent scratching, which could eventually lead to metal leaching into your food.

THE POTS AND PANS YOU'LL NEED I've tried to keep things as easy as possible by using the same pots and pans for all of the recipes in this book. Most of these items are probably in your cupboards already. Here's what you'll need:

Standard loaf pan (9 by 5 inches)

Standard 12-cup muffin tin

10-inch skillet

2 rimmed baking sheets

9-inch square baking dish (preferably glass or enameled bakeware)

9 by 13-inch rectangular pan (preferably glass or enameled bakeware)

5½-quart, or larger, stove top and ovenproof pot with lid (like an enameled Dutch oven)

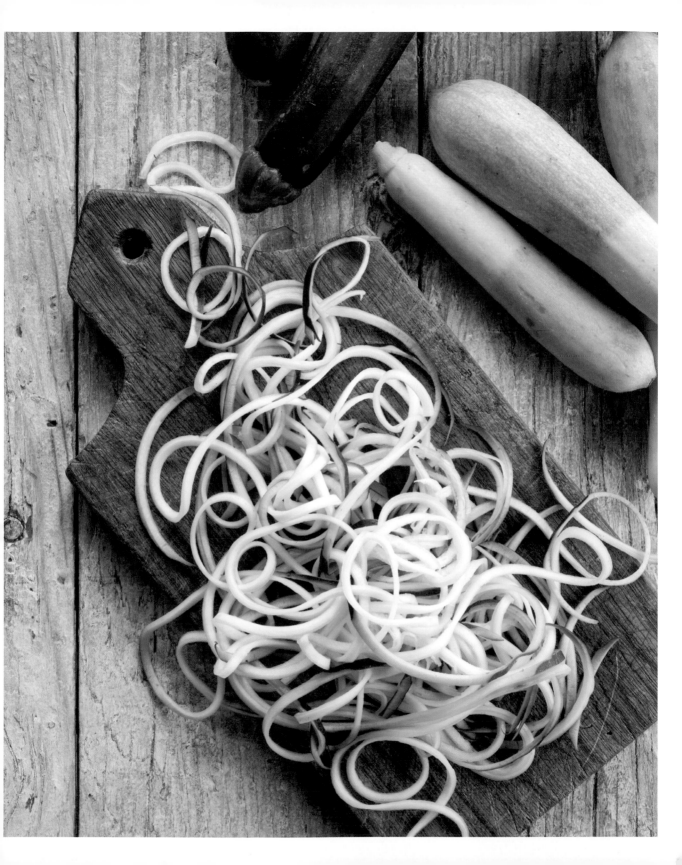

Nut Milk Bag

This fine-mesh bag is used to strain the pulp when making homemade nut or seed milks. Alternatively, you could also use several layers of cheesecloth for a similar straining effect.

Parchment Paper and Baking Cups

Parchment paper and baking cups are an easy alternative to greasing your pans and lining your muffin tins, as they prevent your baked goods from sticking without the need for additional oil or butter. (Parchment is not to be confused with wax paper, which will leave you with a smoky, sticky disaster when baked!) This is one of my favorite baking tools, as it makes the removal of baked goods quick and easy—particularly when removing items from a deep loaf pan or muffin tin.

Salad Shooter

This gadget, which shreds raw vegetables, can cut your prep time in half. I love the texture that shredded vegetables provide to salads, so this tool is invaluable in my kitchen. I use it weekly to prepare all of my salad toppings at once. You can also use shredded vegetables as a rice or pasta substitute.

Silicone Baking Mats and Cups

These nonstick liners are appealing because you can reuse them over and over again, instead of throwing them away after a couple of uses as with parchment paper. (Parchment paper is typically coated with silicone, anyway.) Since silicone mats are relatively new to the market, they haven't been extensively tested for long-term effects, but they are generally considered to not leach chemicals into food and have been deemed safe by the FDA. Use with caution, and do not cut on these mats, as many of them contain a layer of fiberglass to promote even baking.

Spiralizer

This affordable tool is key for quickly creating "noodles" out of your favorite vegetables (see photo on page 33). It typically comes with three blades, which can create angel hair, spaghetti, or ribbonlike "noodles" in just a matter of minutes.

Vegetable Peeler

If you don't want to invest in a spiralizer, a simple vegetable peeler can also be used to create fettuccini-like "noodles" from your favorite veggies. Peelers are available with a julienne blade, too, if you'd like to make spaghetti-like "noodles" or salad toppings by hand.

Whisk

A whisk is a very effective mixing tool when working with dry goods like coconut flour and cocoa powder. It eliminates lumps in a matter of seconds and is essential for making silky-smooth desserts like the Peppermint Fudge Bars (page 166).

HOW TO USE THE RECIPES IN THIS BOOK

The recipes have been labeled according to how they digest, to make detox-friendly meal planning quick and easy. Look for these labels to identify how each recipe combines:

FRESH FRUIT, STARCH, ANIMAL PROTEIN, NUT/SEED/DRIED FRUIT, NEUTRAL, SPECIAL TREAT

Remember to stick to just one category per meal and feel free to enjoy neutral recipes with any category you like. A handful of these recipes are labeled "Special Treats" because they are not perfectly combined, but they all call for whole food ingredients and are included to help make the transition to this healthier lifestyle easier and more enjoyable. For even more properly combined meal-planning guidance, check out the Detox-Friendly Entertaining Menus on page 182.

The recipes in this book are also clearly labeled to accommodate those with food allergies and special dietary needs. Whether you need recipes that are gluten-free, dairy-free, nut-free, soy-free, sugar-free, egg-free, or vegan, there are plenty of options included to make this program work for you.

GF *Gluten-free*   NS *No sugar*

DF *Dairy-free*   EF *Egg-free*

NF *Nut-free*   V   *Vegan*

SF *Soy-free*

MAXIMIZE YOUR KITCHEN SUCCESS

Whether you're a seasoned chef or a cooking newbie, working with new ingredients and healthier cooking techniques can come with a bit of a learning curve. The following tips should help make the transition easier and will ensure that you never have a recipe flop!

- When measuring dry ingredients, always use the "scoop and sweep" method for accurate results: simply dip the measuring cup into the package, scoop a heaping cup of the ingredient, and use the back of a knife to sweep the excess off the top for a level measurement. This is especially important when measuring coconut flour, as even an extra teaspoon may affect the final result.

- When sautéing vegetables, add a splash of water as needed to help prevent sticking, rather than using additional oil or butter.

- When freezing bananas, be sure to peel the bananas before placing them in the freezer, as the peels are very difficult to remove once frozen.

- Many stores now carry prechopped cauliflower and broccoli florets, which can help save on prep time. On average, one 2½-pound head of broccoli or cauliflower is the equivalent of a 2-pound package of chopped florets.

- For recipes that require room-temperature eggs, you can quickly warm refrigerated eggs by placing them in a bowl filled with hot (not boiling) tap water while you prepare the rest of the recipe.

- When working with salad dressings and dips, feel free to replace the dried herbs with fresh herbs, and vice versa. Always use a ratio of 1 part dried herbs to 3 parts fresh herbs (for example, 1 teaspoon dried herbs = 1 tablespoon fresh herbs).

- Depending on the temperature of your kitchen, your coconut oil may or may not be in liquid form. If you need to melt solidified coconut oil, you can place it in an ovenproof bowl and warm it on top of a preheating oven or even place it directly in the oven for faster results. (Be careful when removing the melted oil—you don't want to spill any type of oil in an oven and risk grease fires.)

- In recipes that call for coconut flour, I don't recommend making any substitutions, unless otherwise noted in the directions. Real eggs and liquid sweeteners are essential in these grain-free recipes, and even the smallest change might affect your results. Experiment at your own risk!

Remember, practice makes perfect, and you'll be a pro at whipping up healthy meals in no time. The recipes in this book can be easily customized to suit your taste, so don't be afraid to get creative and adapt the ingredients as you see fit. You're going to love eating this way and how you look and feel even more, so let's get cooking!

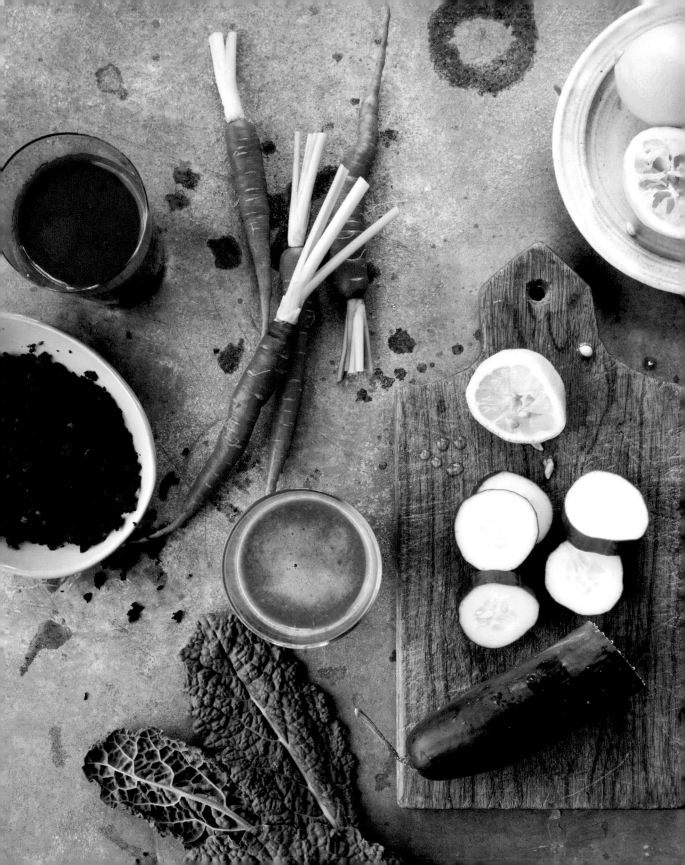

liquid nourishment

Juices and smoothies are ideal ways to start your morning, since they are bursting with nutrition and set a healthy tone for the rest of your day. Blending and juicing vegetables allows us to consume more fresh produce than we would otherwise, because they often pack several fruits and vegetables into a single glass, making it easy to meet our daily requirements. If you're skeptical about adding leafy greens to your juices and smoothies, I urge you to give it a try—you may be surprised to find that you mostly taste the fruit, not the greens! A quick and convenient option for folks on the go, the following recipes can be whipped up in minutes and sipped through a straw during your busy mornings.

kale lemonade

NEUTRAL | (GF) (DF) (NF) (SF) (EF) (V) | *Serves 1*

This sweet and tart juice is the perfect way to sneak an extra dose of green veggies into your day. Kale is a nutritional powerhouse, loaded with antioxidants like vitamins A, C, and K, and by juicing it, you can benefit from this leafy green while also avoiding its famously fibrous texture. Any variety of kale will work for this recipe, but I prefer to use Lacinato kale (also known as Dino kale), as it seems to produce the most juice. (Pictured on page 41.)

5 kale leaves

1 cucumber

1 Fuji apple

½ lemon

Feed all of the ingredients into the mouth of a juicer, extracting the juice from the pulp. Pour the juice into a glass and enjoy immediately.

NOTE: *If using a centrifugal juicer with more than one speed, juice softer produce, like leafy greens, on the low setting for best juice extraction. Firmer fruits and veggies, like carrots, apples, and lemons, will require the high setting, which can typically handle apple cores and lemon peels effortlessly.*

cucumber lime cooler

NEUTRAL | (GF) (DF) (NF) (SF) (EF) (V) | *Serves 1*

This cooling juice is perfect for a quick pick-me-up, as cucumbers are a great source of B vitamins and electrolytes. Combined with the vitamins and antioxidants from the addition of celery, parsley, and pear, this juice may help reduce inflammation in the body and will leave you feeling calm and refreshed for the rest of the morning. (Pictured on page 41.)

1 cucumber

2 celery stalks

Handful of fresh
  parsley

1 ripe pear

½ lime

Feed all of the ingredients into the mouth of a juicer, extracting the juice from the pulp. Pour the juice into a glass and enjoy immediately.

NOTE: *For best nutrient absorption, drink your juice slowly, swishing it around in your mouth, so your saliva can properly begin the digestive process.*

JUICES VERSUS SMOOTHIES There is usually a bit of confusion surrounding juices and smoothies, so let's briefly discuss the difference between the two.

A juicer removes the pulp and fiber from fresh produce, leaving you with pure liquid nourishment that can be absorbed very quickly by the body. In a way, juicing extends the evening fast between your dinner the previous night and your first meal of the day, because the digestive system isn't activated until you eat something heavier. Juices contain no fiber, making them less filling than smoothies, but they are perfect for those who do not have much of an appetite in the morning—particularly those who drink coffee all morning long instead of having breakfast. You may soon find that fresh vegetable juice provides you with a natural boost of energy, without the need for caffeine.

Blending, on the other hand, pulverizes whole fruits and vegetables without removing the pulp, creating a thick, smooth beverage that is more filling than juice. The body doesn't assimilate smoothies as quickly as juices, but they are still easier to digest than a traditional breakfast, since the blender has already "chewed up" the food for you. They are also perfect for those who crave fruitier beverages, as the inclusion of fiber helps balance the body's absorption of the natural fruit sugars.

Both juices and smoothies can play an important role in an overall healthy diet, so whether you choose to consume one or the other, or both, is completely up to your discretion. Be sure to enjoy these nutritious drinks on an empty stomach for best nutrient absorption and assimilation.

back to your roots

NEUTRAL | GF DF NF SF EF V | *Serves 1*

This deeply red juice features sweet carrots, earthy beets, and a touch of warming ginger to get your blood pumping. Beets have a reputation for cleansing the liver, but recent studies suggest that nitrate-rich beet juice may also improve cardiovascular health and exercise performance,[1] while also significantly reducing blood pressure.[2] Paired with the beta-carotene and vitamins A, B, and E in carrots, this naturally sweet juice looks as vibrant as it will make you feel.

4 large carrots

1 large beet

1 green apple

1 (1-inch) knob ginger

Feed all of the ingredients into the mouth of a juicer, extracting the juice from the pulp. Pour the juice into a glass and enjoy immediately.

NOTE: *There's no need to peel any of your ingredients—the juicer will do all of the work for you.*

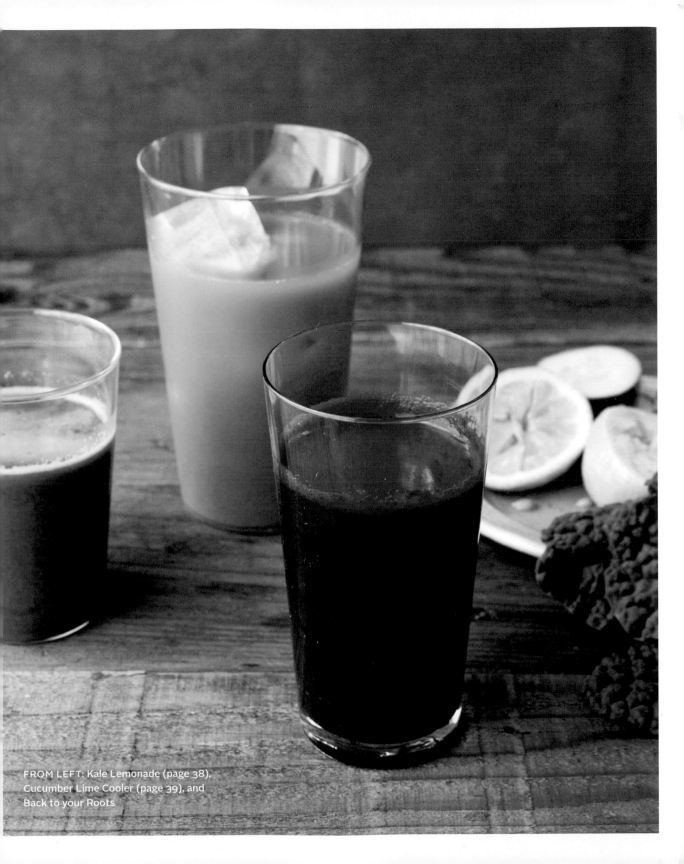

FROM LEFT: Kale Lemonade (page 38), Cucumber Lime Cooler (page 39), and Back to your Roots

V-6 juice

NEUTRAL | (GF) (DF) (NF) (SF) (NS) (EF) (V) | *Serves 1*

This juice is sure to rev your engine, packing several servings of vegetables into a single glass. Unlike store-bought vegetable juice, this homemade version is unpasteurized and free of added salt or preservatives, providing a more refreshing flavor and even more nutrition. As with any juice, the flavor can be customized to suit your taste, so feel free to add more carrots for a sweeter juice, or more celery for a natural boost of salt.

2 celery stalks

1 ripe tomato

2 large carrots

½ red bell pepper

½ cucumber

Small handful fresh parsley

1 lime

Feed all of the ingredients into the mouth of a juicer, extracting the juice from the pulp. Pour the juice into a glass and enjoy immediately.

banana nut protein shake

NUT/SEED/DRIED FRUIT | GF DF SF EF V | *Serves 1*

All of the flavors you love in a banana nut muffin are served up in this cold and creamy smoothie. Hemp hearts are the tender center of the hemp seed, featuring all of the essential amino acids necessary for building protein in the body. Unlike flax seeds, which you need to grind ahead of time to benefit from their full nutritional profile, hemp hearts can be enjoyed directly from the bag over a salad or blended seamlessly into a smoothie. Paired with frozen banana, raw walnuts, and a couple of handfuls of fresh spinach (don't worry, you can't taste it!), you can count on this delicious shake to leave you feeling full and satisfied all morning long.

1 cup Homemade Almond Milk (page 178)

2 tablespoons hemp hearts

Small handful of raw walnuts (about ¼ cup)

2 handfuls fresh baby spinach leaves

1 frozen banana

½ teaspoon ground cinnamon

½ teaspoon vanilla extract (optional)

1 handful ice cubes (optional)

Combine all of the ingredients in a high-speed blender and blend until completely smooth. Pour into a glass and serve immediately.

NOTE: *The addition of vanilla extract can make a smoothie taste truly gourmet, but unless otherwise labeled, it does contain a small amount of alcohol. Alcohol free vanilla flavor is also widely available and can be used interchangeably in any recipe, if you prefer.*

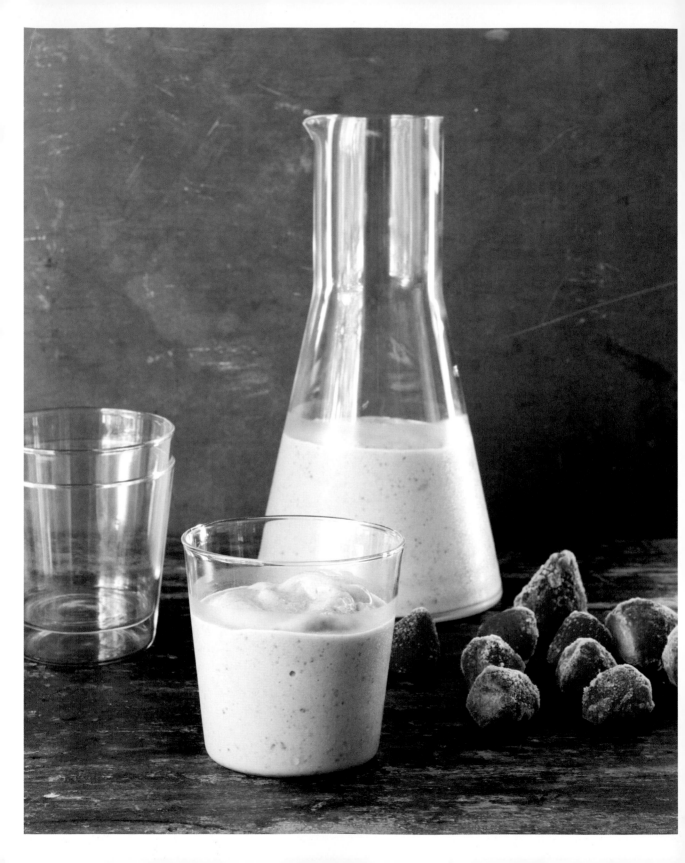

strawberry basil blast

FRESH FRUIT | GF DF SF EF V | *Serves 1*

Fresh basil enhances the naturally sweet flavor of strawberries in this tasty shake, which is loaded with antioxidants that may help improve blood sugar regulation and reduce inflammation in the body. The addition of avocado provides a creamy texture and helps the body absorb fat-soluble vitamins, making for a truly satiating shake. This unexpected flavor combination may soon become one of your favorite morning drinks.

1½ cups whole frozen strawberries (about 6 ounces)

1 cup Homemade Almond Milk (page 178)

1 tablespoon fresh minced basil

¼ small ripe avocado, pitted

3 soft Medjool dates, pitted

1 tablespoon freshly squeezed lemon juice

Combine all of the ingredients in a high-speed blender and blend until completely smooth and creamy. Serve immediately.

NOTE: *When making green smoothies without a high-speed blender, blend together the leafy greens and liquid first, to help break down the greens completely, then add in the rest of the ingredients and blend again. The smoother you can blend these drinks, the more enjoyable they will be!*

tropical twister

FRESH FRUIT | GF DF NF SF EF V | *Serves 1*

You don't need to be near a beach to enjoy a taste of the tropics. Pineapple and mango provide a full dose of vitamin C for the day, along with a hefty dose of enzymes, which may help boost digestion. Paired with a ripe avocado, which adds healthy fat and a creamy texture, and fresh lime juice, this smoothie is sure to make your morning look brighter. (Pictured on page 50.)

1 cup coconut water

¼ small ripe avocado, pitted

1 handful fresh spinach

½ cup frozen pineapple chunks

½ cup frozen mango chunks

½ frozen banana

1 tablespoon freshly squeezed lime juice

Combine all of the ingredients in a high-speed blender and blend until completely smooth. Serve immediately.

NOTE: *You can always find coconut water inside a freshly opened young Thai coconut, but coconut water is now more available and convenient than ever with many packaged varieties available at your local grocery store. For the best taste and quality, try the raw and organic coconut water from Harmless Harvest or Exotic Superfoods (see Resources, page 184).*

ROTATE YOUR GREENS Most of the green smoothies in this book call for spinach, because its mild taste blends seamlessly into any fruit smoothie without affecting the flavor. Once you've started to enjoy green smoothies on a regular basis, try rotating the leafy greens you use for the greatest variety of nutrition. Romaine, kale, bok choy, collard greens, parsley, mustard greens, dandelion greens, beet greens, and more are all great options, so get adventurous!

blended apple pie à la mode

FRESH FRUIT | GF DF SF EF V | *Serves 1*

The name says it all—this smoothie tastes like a slice of apple pie blended together with a scoop of ice cream! Ripe avocado provides this shake's creamy texture, along with a serving of healthy fat, while the dates add the sweetness of pie with a hefty dose of fiber and minerals, including iron, potassium, and magnesium. Who says you can't have pie for breakfast?

1 cup Homemade Almond Milk (page 178)

¼ small ripe avocado, pitted

1 Fuji apple, cored and sliced

3 soft Medjool dates, pitted

½ teaspoon ground cinnamon

½ teaspoon vanilla extract

A handful of ice cubes (optional)

Combine all of the ingredients in a high-powered blender and blend until smooth and creamy. Serve immediately.

NOTE: *For a burst of nutrition, try adding a handful of fresh baby spinach to this shake. It will give you an extra serving of greens for the day, without affecting the apple pie flavor.*

chocolate chia shake

NUT/SEED/DRIED FRUIT | GF DF SF EF V | *Serves 1*

Though it looks and tastes like a thick, chocolate milk shake, this smoothie is brimming with fiber, calcium, and omega-3 fatty acids, thanks to the addition of chia seeds. These tiny seeds pack a wallop of protein for their size and also provide this shake with a thick texture, as they expand when added to liquid. Paired with frozen bananas, which become quite ice cream-like when blended, and fiber-rich dates, this shake tastes as indulgent as it looks.

1 cup Homemade Almond Milk (page 178)

1 tablespoon chia seeds

2 soft Medjool dates, pitted

2 tablespoons raw cacao powder or cocoa powder

1 frozen banana

¼ teaspoon vanilla extract

2 or 3 ice cubes

1. Combine the almond milk, chia seeds, and dates in a high-speed blender and blend until the chia seeds and dates are completely broken down.

2. Add the raw cacao powder, banana, vanilla, and ice cubes and blend again, until thick and creamy. Serve immediately.

NOTE: *If dates are difficult to find, 1 tablespoon of maple syrup can be used instead.*

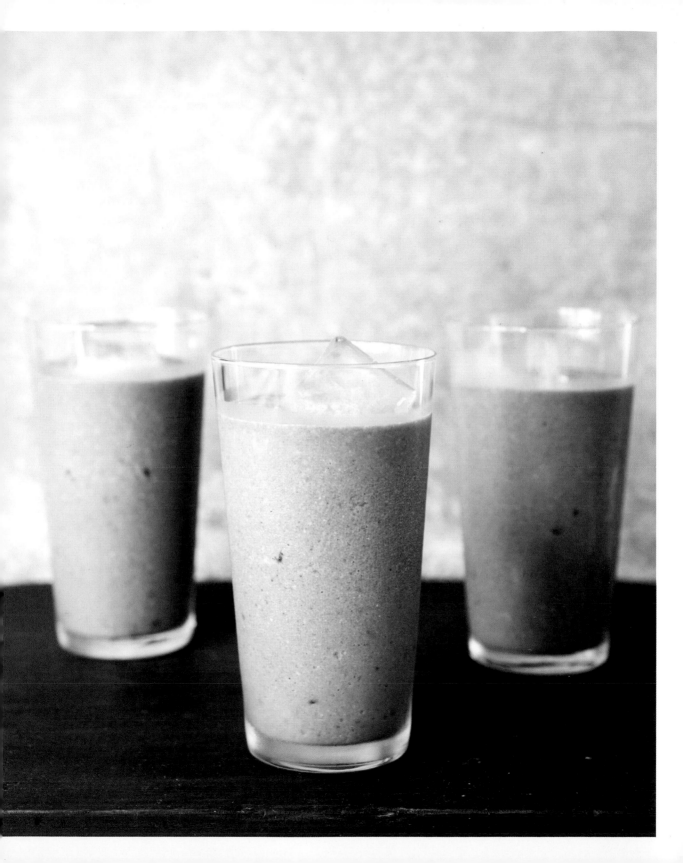

FROM LEFT: Peachy Green Cleanser and
Tropical Twister (page 46)

peachy green cleanser

FRESH FRUIT | GF DF SF EF V | *Serves 1*

More than just a garnish, parsley is a powerful herb that contains important vitamins and flavonoids, which may help reduce the risk of certain cancers and inflammation in the body. Parsley is also a natural diuretic, helping increase the flow of fluids through the kidneys, which has given it a reputation as a kidney cleanser. Lightly sweetened with frozen peaches, pineapple, and dates, parsley is the star of this show, creating a uniquely clean and fresh-tasting smoothie.

1 cup Homemade Almond Milk (page 178)

1 cup frozen peaches

½ cup frozen pineapple chunks

Small handful fresh parsley

2 soft Medjool dates, pitted

Combine all of the ingredients in a high-speed blender and blend until completely smooth. Pour into a glass and serve immediately.

NOTE: *When first using parsley, you may want to start off with just a small amount to help get your body acclimated to its cleansing properties. Headaches can occur as a side effect of eating this potent herb, but they typically diminish once your body becomes accustomed to its unique compounds.*

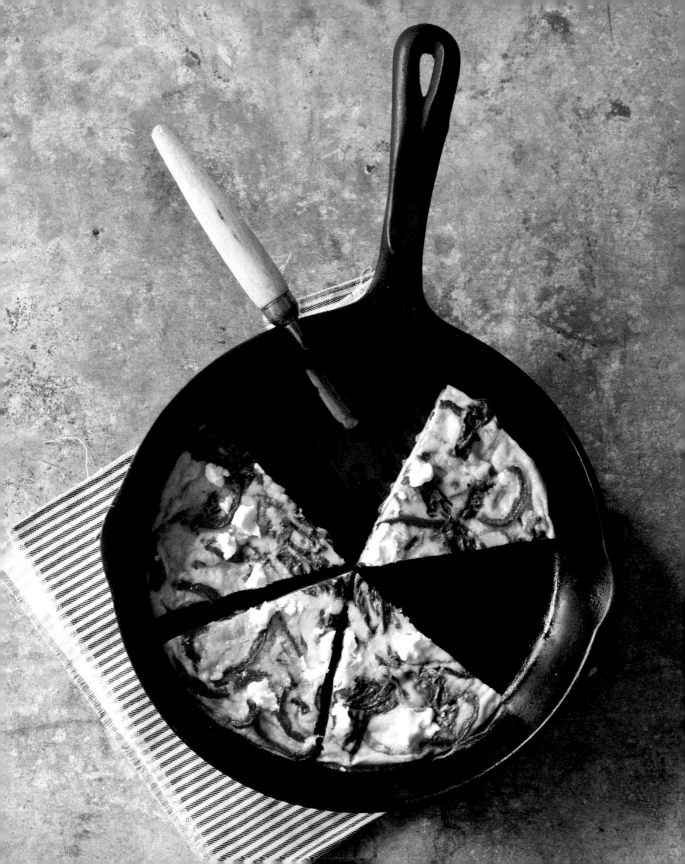

morning favorites

CHAPTER 4

Though juices and smoothies tend to be the foundation of a detox-friendly morning, the following recipes are included for days when liquid nourishment just isn't enough. With options like Overnight Chia Pudding (page 59) for a quick breakfast on the go, Maple Pecan Granola (page 54) to satisfy your cereal cravings, and Blender Banana Pancakes (page 68) for an easy weekend brunch, you're sure to enjoy everything you eat while still working toward your health goals.

maple pecan granola

NUT/SEED/DRIED FRUIT | (GF) (DF) (SF) (EF) (V) | *Serves 4*

It's hard to believe that this granola is grain-free, as it sticks together just like the traditional versions, without the use of butter, oil, or refined sugar. Instead, it's naturally sweetened with pure maple syrup, which provides essential minerals like iron, calcium, zinc, manganese, and potassium, along with its distinct maple flavor. Paired with crunchy pecans and shredded coconut, this morning treat will soon become a weekend favorite.

1 cup pecans

1 cup shredded unsweetened coconut

½ cup hulled sunflower seeds

¼ cup maple syrup

1 teaspoon vanilla extract

2 teaspoons ground cinnamon

⅛ teaspoon sea salt

Homemade Almond Milk (page 178), for serving (optional)

Sliced banana or raisins, for topping (optional)

1. Preheat the oven to 250°F and line a large baking sheet with parchment paper or a silicone liner.

2. Place the pecans in a food processor fitted with an "S" blade and briefly pulse, just enough to break the pecans down into smaller pieces, leaving a few chunks for texture.

3. Transfer the pecan pieces to a bowl and add the coconut, sunflower seeds, maple syrup, vanilla, cinnamon, and salt. Stir well to combine. Spread out the mixture evenly on the lined baking sheet, using your hands to press the granola into a thin, uniform layer.

4. Bake for 30 minutes, rotating the pan halfway through the baking time to ensure even toasting. The final granola should be lightly golden. Remove from the oven and allow the granola to cool and harden completely in the pan.

5. Break the granola into pieces and serve with homemade almond milk and a topping of sliced banana or raisins. Leftover granola can be stored at room temperature for up to 3 days, or in the refrigerator for up to 2 weeks.

NOTE: *Baking this granola at a low temperature keeps its delicate oils intact and helps prevent the formation of acrylamide, a harmful carcinogen (see page 22).*

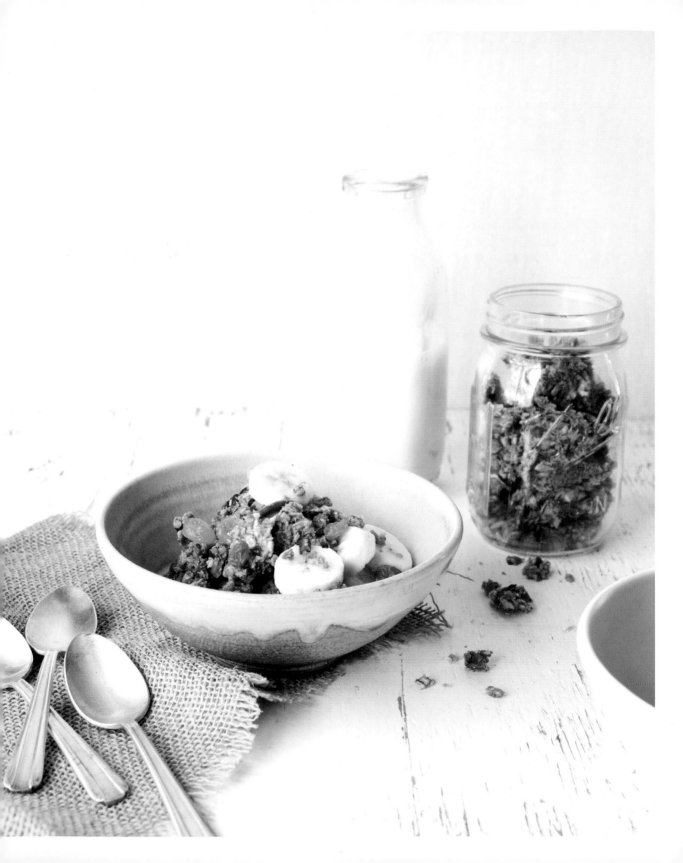

banana coconut muffins

NUT/SEED/DRIED FRUIT | (GF) (DF) (NF) (SF) (EF) (V) | *Makes 12 muffins*

It's rare to find a coconut flour recipe that comes together without the use of eggs, but that's what makes these muffins so special—they're not only egg-free, but also naturally sweetened using only ripe bananas! Unlike traditional baked goods, these muffins won't rise when baked, but despite their moist and dense texture, they are surprisingly light, thanks to the fluffy nature of coconut flour. Be sure to use bananas with lots of brown spots on their skin for best flavor.

⅔ cup coconut flour

3 cups mashed very ripe bananas (about 6 large bananas)

1 tablespoon ground cinnamon

1 cup shredded unsweetened coconut

2 teaspoons vanilla extract

1 teaspoon baking soda

2 teaspoons raw apple cider vinegar

1. Preheat the oven to 350°F and line a standard muffin tin with parchment baking cups.

2. In a large bowl, stir together the coconut flour and mashed banana until well combined, then add in the cinnamon, coconut, vanilla, and baking soda. Stir until a thick, uniform batter is formed, then quickly stir in the raw apple cider vinegar.

3. Divide the batter among the 12 muffin cups, keeping in mind that these muffins will not rise with baking. Bake for 30 to 35 minutes, until the muffin tops are slightly golden and firm to the touch. Allow the muffins to cool before serving and store the leftovers in a sealed container at room temperature for up to 3 days, or in the refrigerator for up to 1 week.

NOTE: *Certain fruits, including bananas, apples, and tomatoes, produce ethylene gas, which naturally induces ripening. Place unripe bananas in a bag with an apple or a tomato to trap these gases and speed up the ripening process.*

buckwheat banana bread

SPECIAL TREAT | (GF) (DF) (NF) (SF) (EF) | *Makes 1 (9 by 5-inch) loaf*

This dense and hearty loaf features nutrient-rich buckwheat (see page 22), a gluten-free pseudograin that is actually a fruit seed but behaves similarly to a grain. Paired with ripe bananas, honey, and cinnamon, it creates a nutty, lightly sweetened quick bread without the use of eggs or excess sugar. For best flavor and appearance, make your own buckwheat flour by simply grinding raw buckwheat groats in a high-speed blender or coffee grinder. Though buckwheat is technically a seed, it is often considered a grain for food-combining purposes, as are other pseudograins like quinoa and amaranth. Use your own discretion when choosing how you best digest these protein-rich seeds.

1 cup buckwheat flour

1½ cups mashed ripe bananas (about 3 large bananas)

2 teaspoons ground cinnamon

¼ cup melted coconut oil, plus more for serving (optional)

¼ teaspoon sea salt

1 teaspoon vanilla extract

⅓ cup honey

1 teaspoon baking soda

1 tablespoon raw apple cider vinegar

Butter, for serving (optional)

1. Preheat the oven to 350°F and grease a standard loaf pan generously with coconut oil or, for even easier removal later, line it with parchment paper.

2. In a large mixing bowl, stir together the buckwheat flour, bananas, and cinnamon, followed by the melted coconut oil, salt, vanilla, honey, baking soda, and vinegar.

3. Pour the batter into the greased loaf pan and smooth the top with a spatula.

4. Bake for 35 minutes, or until the center of the loaf is firm and the top has begun to crack. Allow the bread to cool in the pan for 20 minutes and then flip it out onto a wire rack to cool completely.

5. Slice and serve with a pat of butter or coconut oil, if desired.

make it vegan Replace the honey with ⅓ cup maple syrup.

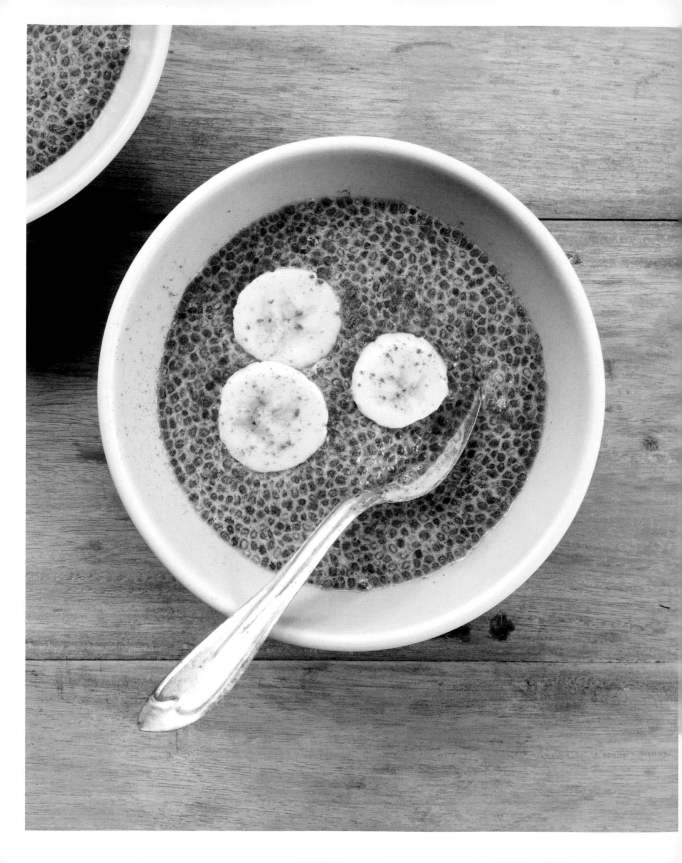

overnight chia pudding

NUT/SEED/DRIED FRUIT | GF DF SF EF V | *Serves 4*

This tapioca-like pudding makes the perfect breakfast for a person on the go. It can be prepared in just a matter of minutes and thickens overnight in the refrigerator for a breakfast that is ready to grab on your way out the door. Chia seeds are not only filling, thanks to their hefty fiber content, but also packed with omega-3 fatty acids, which are important for brain health. Talk about a smart way to start your day!

¾ cup chia seeds

4 cups Homemade Almond Milk (page 178)

¼ cup maple syrup

2 teaspoons vanilla extract

2 teaspoons ground cinnamon

Sliced banana, for topping (optional)

1. Combine the chia seeds, almond milk, maple syrup, vanilla, and cinnamon in a large bowl and whisk together. (Using a whisk helps prevent the seeds from clumping together.)

2. Divide the mixture between four glass containers with lids and place them in the refrigerator to set overnight.

3. Enjoy chilled, with slices of banana on top. Extra pudding can be stored in an airtight container in the refrigerator for up to 4 days.

make it sugar-free Replace the maple syrup with stevia, to taste.

cinnamon coffee cake with macaroon crumble

SPECIAL TREAT | **GF** **DF** **NF** **SF** | *Makes 1 (9-inch square) cake*

This soft and spongy coffee cake is made with coconut flour for a fiber-rich and gluten-free alternative to serve at Sunday brunch. Don't fear the large number of eggs called for—they give this cake structure but do not impart an "eggy" taste or texture. Though this cake is naturally sweetened with honey and applesauce, it is surprisingly similar to a cake made with wheat flour and refined sugar. The macaroon crumble also makes for a more traditional-looking coffee cake, without the need for copious amounts of brown sugar on top.

CAKE

¾ cup coconut flour

6 eggs, at room temperature

¾ cup unsweetened applesauce

2 tablespoons ground cinnamon

½ cup honey

1 teaspoon baking soda

MACAROON CRUMBLE

⅔ cup shredded unsweetened coconut

2 tablespoons maple syrup

Pinch of salt

1. Preheat the oven to 350°F and line a 9-inch square baking dish with parchment paper.

2. Prepare the cake: In a large bowl, combine the coconut flour, eggs, applesauce, cinnamon, honey, and baking soda and whisk well, breaking up any lumps in the batter. It will most likely be thicker than traditional cake batter, particularly if any of the ingredients you use are cold, but it will still bake properly.

3. Transfer the batter to the lined baking dish and use a spatula to spread it evenly toward the edges. Smooth the top and then set aside while you prepare the crumble.

4. Prepare the macaroon crumble: Place the shredded coconut, maple syrup, and salt in a small food processor and process until the coconut mixture starts to stick together. Use your hands to sprinkle the sticky mixture over the top of the cake and then gently press the crumble into the top of the cake.

5. Bake for 35 to 40 minutes, until the center is firm and the edges are golden. Allow to cool for 15 minutes before cutting and serving.

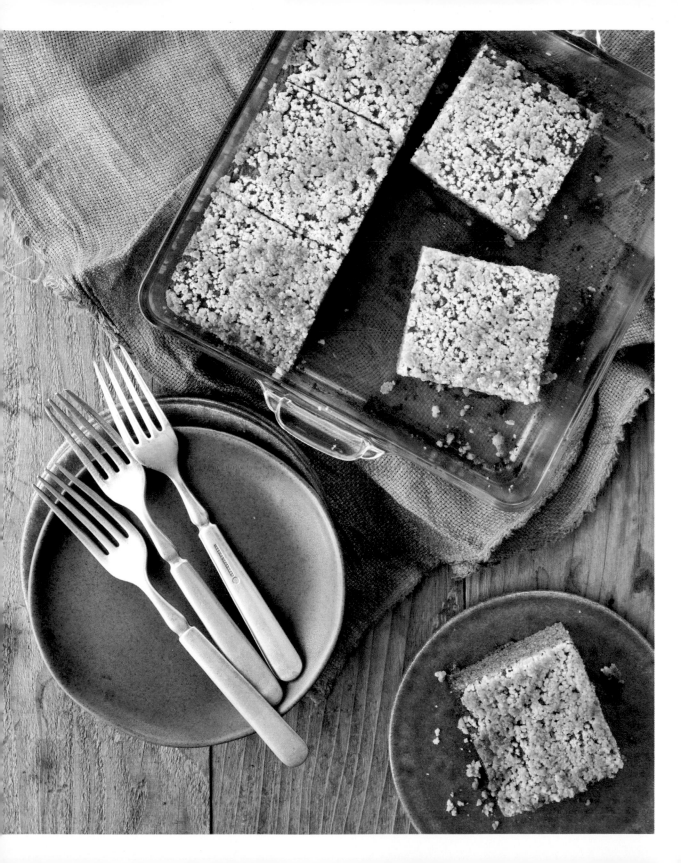

eggs benedict with healthy hollandaise

ANIMAL PROTEIN | (GF) (NF) (SF) (NS) | *Serves 4*

Traditional hollandaise sauce is heavy and overwhelming to prepare, typically calling for several raw egg yolks, not to mention an entire stick of butter. This lighter alternative calls for just a touch of grass-fed butter, which is rich in vitamin A, to help emulsify this smooth and velvety cauliflower-based sauce. Served over warm eggplant, which becomes slightly breadlike when broiled, and topped with a sliced ripe tomato, this version tastes just as decadent as the original, while being easier on your digestion. If you don't care for eggplant, feel free to use any other favorite nonstarchy vegetables as a base for this dish, such as sautéed spinach, asparagus, or zucchini.

8 (½-inch-wide) eggplant slices

Sea salt

8 (½-inch-wide) ripe tomato slices

1 teaspoon raw apple cider vinegar (optional)

8 eggs

HEALTHY HOLLANDAISE

2 cups chopped cauliflower florets

¼ cup water

¼ teaspoon sea salt

1 tablespoon freshly squeezed lemon juice

1 tablespoon nutritional yeast

1 tablespoon grass-fed butter

1. Place the eggplant in a large bowl and sprinkle generously with sea salt. Use your hands to rub the salt evenly over the eggplant slices, then set aside and allow them to sweat for 30 minutes. This removes their excess moisture and bitterness.

2. Prepare the hollandaise: In a small saucepan filled with 1 inch of water and fitted with a steam basket, steam the cauliflower florets until they are very tender, 10 to 12 minutes. Transfer the steamed cauliflower to a blender and add in the water, salt, lemon juice, nutritional yeast, and butter. Blend until completely smooth, then set aside.

3. When the eggplant has sufficiently sweated, rinse the slices with water and pat dry with a towel. Turn on the oven broiler and arrange the eggplant slices in a single layer on a baking sheet. Broil the slices for 5 to 7 minutes on each side, until lightly golden. Transfer the cooked eggplant to a serving plate and top each piece with a tomato slice. Set aside while you prepare the eggs. (You can place the slices in a warm oven, if you like.)

4. Fill a shallow saucepan with a few inches of water and the vinegar (vinegar helps egg whites set, but it does add a slight flavor to the cooked eggs, so feel free to leave it out if you prefer) and bring it to nearly boiling, then reduce the heat slightly. (You should see tiny bubbles forming on the bottom of the pan.) Working with one egg at a time, crack an egg into a small dish, then bring the dish to the surface of the hot water and carefully pour the egg into the saucepan. Use a spoon to nudge the egg whites closer to the yolks to help keep the egg together while it cooks. Cover and allow the eggs to cook until the whites are set, about 5 minutes. (Feel free to cook longer if you prefer a less runny yolk.) Use a slotted spoon to remove the cooked eggs. (Alternatively, you can skip the poaching process and panfry the eggs instead.)

5. Arrange each cooked egg over a slice of warm eggplant and sliced tomato and then top with a generous spoonful of hollandaise sauce. Serve immediately.

make it omnivore-friendly Add your favorite high-quality meat to this properly combined dish.

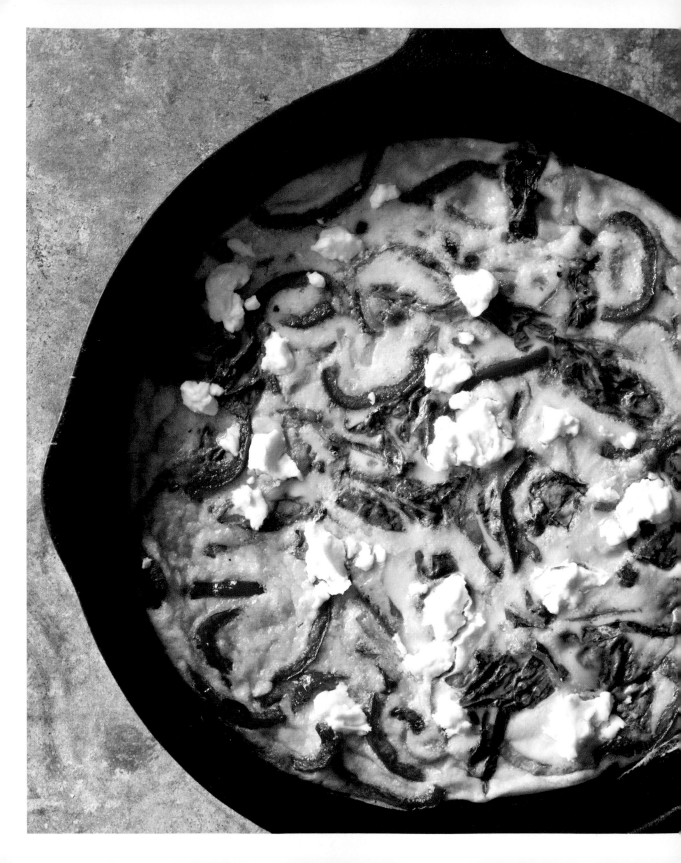

caramelized onion & red bell pepper frittata

ANIMAL PROTEIN | (GF) (NF) (SF) (NS) | *Serves 4 to 6*

I love that frittatas are quicker to make than omelets and can easily serve a group of people in less time than it would take to prepare eggs individually to order. Be sure to use a skillet that is ovenproof so that it can go directly from stove top to oven without the need to dirty an extra dish. Feel free to enjoy this filling and protein-rich meal at any time of the day.

1 tablespoon butter

½ yellow onion, thinly sliced

1 red bell pepper, cored, seeded, and chopped

1 cup fresh baby spinach

8 eggs

¼ teaspoon sea salt

2 ounces chèvre (soft goat cheese)

1. Preheat the oven to 400°F.

2. Melt the butter in an ovenproof skillet over medium heat. Add the onion and sauté until tender and golden, 8 to 10 minutes. Add the bell pepper and sauté for another 5 minutes. Add the spinach and cook for another minute, until just wilted.

3. Crack the eggs into a large bowl, add the salt, and beat well with a fork. Pour the beaten eggs into the skillet and use the fork to press the vegetables down into the egg mixture so that the eggs cover the veggies completely. Crumble the chèvre over the top, then place the pan in the oven and bake until the top is set and lightly golden, 10 to 15 minutes.

4. Cut into wedges and serve warm.

DON'T DITCH THE YOLKS! Though egg yolks have been vilified over the years, recent research shows that consuming whole eggs does not increase the risk of heart attack or stroke, and those who ate more eggs actually had a reduced risk of stroke.[1] Cholesterol is essential to the human body, which is why our liver produces it if we don't get enough from dietary sources. By eating cholesterol, the body actually has to produce less. Almost all of the nutrients in eggs are contained in the yolk, including B vitamins and choline, which are essential for healthy brain function, and antioxidants like lutein and zeaxanthin, which are thought to promote eye health. So, by eating the whole egg, you'll enjoy more nutritional bang for your buck and feel satisfied long after your meal.

no-bake coconut granola bars

NUT/SEED/DRIED FRUIT | (GF) (DF) (NF) (SF) (EF) (V) | *Makes 12 bars*

These granola bars are free of grains and added oils, making them healthier than any store-bought bar, but just as convenient, as they can be stored at room temperature. Since many schools and airplanes are now nut-free, these coconut-based bars also make the perfect allergy-friendly snack to send off with your loved ones. Once you get the process down, feel free to use any combination of nuts, seeds, and spices that you like to create your own customized bar.

1½ cups shredded unsweetened coconut

¾ cup hulled sunflower seeds

¼ cup hemp hearts

½ teaspoon sea salt

½ cup maple syrup

1. Line a 9-inch square pan with parchment paper and set aside.

2. Combine the coconut, sunflower seeds, hemp hearts, and salt in a large bowl and stir well to mix.

3. In a small saucepan over medium-low heat, bring the maple syrup to a boil. The moment the edge of the maple syrup starts to bubble, set a timer and allow it to boil for 3 to 4 minutes, without stirring, until it turns slightly more golden in color. Immediately pour the boiled maple syrup over the coconut mixture and stir very well to coat evenly.

4. Transfer the sticky mixture to the lined pan, and use your hands to press the mixture evenly into the pan. Use an extra piece of parchment paper on top to keep your hands clean. Press firmly to really pack the mixture together well.

5. Place in the freezer to cool quickly for about 30 minutes, and then remove and allow the bars to come to room temperature. Use a sharp knife to slice 12 bars and store them in a sealed container at room temperature for up to 1 week or in the freezer for up to 2 months.

NOTE: *Though the FDA recognizes coconut as a tree nut, the American College of Allergy, Asthma & Immunology classifies coconut as a fruit, not a botanical nut, and has stated that most people who are allergic to tree nuts can safely eat coconut.[2] If you are allergic to tree nuts, be sure to talk to your allergist before adding coconut to your diet.*

cinnamon raisin snack bars

NUT/SEED/DRIED FRUIT | (GF) (DF) (SF) (EF) (V) | *Makes 6 to 8 bars*

These fiber-rich bars are quick and easy to prepare and are an affordable way to snack without relying on the expensive store-bought variety. Raisins are a good source of calcium and iron and may help prevent constipation, while walnuts are loaded with vitamin E, which may support heart health. A healthy dose of cinnamon makes these bars taste like a cinnamon raisin cookie, and as an added bonus, it may help balance your blood sugar at the same time.

1 cup raisins

1 cup raw walnuts

1 cup shredded unsweetened coconut

1 teaspoon ground cinnamon

¼ teaspoon sea salt

1. Line a standard loaf pan with parchment paper (or, for thinner bars, use a 9-inch square pan).

2. In a large food processor fitted with an "S" blade, process the raisins until they start to stick together in a ball.

3. Add the walnuts, coconut, cinnamon, and salt and process again until a somewhat uniform dough is created that sticks together when pressed between your fingers.

4. Transfer the mixture to the prepared pan and use your hands to press the dough firmly and evenly into the bottom of the pan, using another piece of parchment paper on top to keep your hands clean.

5. Place the pan in the freezer to set for 1 hour and then slice into 6 to 8 bars. Store the bars in an airtight container in the refrigerator for up to 1 week or in the freezer for up to 2 months.

blender banana pancakes

SPECIAL TREAT | (GF) (NF) (SF) | *Serves 2*

These moist and fluffy pancakes feature ripe bananas and fiber-rich coconut flour but taste surprisingly authentic when panfried in a greased skillet. With two whole eggs per serving, these pancakes are loaded with protein, which will help balance your blood sugar if you choose to enjoy them with a splash of pure maple syrup. Keep in mind that the ripeness of your bananas will determine how sweet your pancakes are, so for sweeter pancakes with a stronger banana flavor, use bananas with lots of brown spots on their skin, and use bananas with less spots for a more neutral flavor.

2 ripe bananas, mashed (about 1 cup)

4 eggs

5 level tablespoons coconut flour

½ teaspoon baking soda

½ teaspoon vanilla extract

Pinch of sea salt

Coconut oil or butter, for panfrying

Maple syrup, for serving (optional)

1. Combine the bananas, eggs, coconut flour, baking soda, vanilla, and salt in a high-speed blender and blend until completely smooth.

2. Melt the coconut oil in a skillet over medium heat and pour the batter into the hot skillet, using about ¼ cup of batter for each pancake. Use the measuring cup or the back of a spoon to spread out the batter a bit, creating a pancake approximately 4 inches in diameter.

3. Cook for 4 to 5 minutes, until the edges are firm, then flip and cook for another 2 to 3 minutes, until the pancake is cooked through. Repeat with the remaining batter, then serve warm with maple syrup.

NOTE: *This recipe can easily be doubled or tripled to accommodate the number of people in your household.*

make it dairy-free Use coconut oil instead of butter for panfrying.

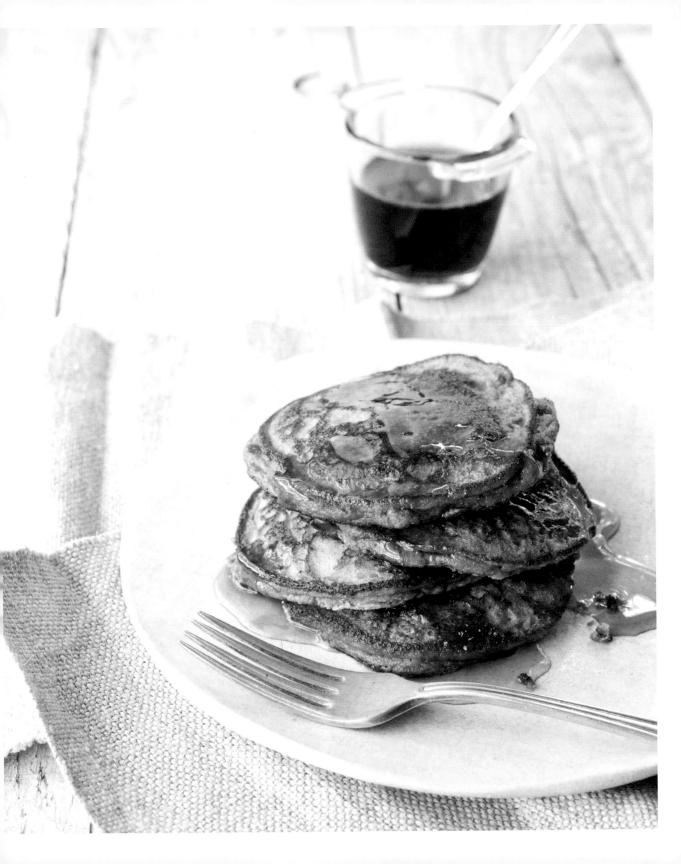

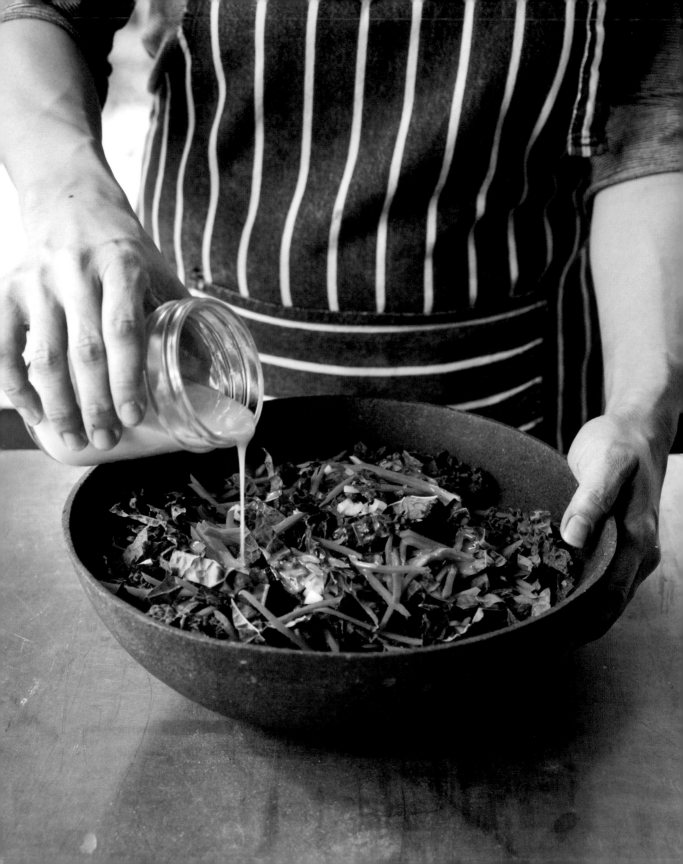

salads, dressings & sides

No one wants to live off of boring side salads or bland steamed vegetables, and luckily, you don't have to. The following recipes include hearty portions and loads of flavor, which will make eating your vegetables an absolute pleasure. Keep in mind that a salad will taste only as good as its ingredients, so be sure to look for fresh and in-season produce as often as possible and don't be afraid to make substitutions accordingly. To make life easier, try making one or two batches of salad dressing at the beginning of the week so that they are ready for a convenient meal that can be prepared faster than visiting a drive-through window. Once you taste these delicious dressings and dips, you may suddenly find yourself craving more vegetables!

creamy jalapeño dressing

NUT/SEED/DRIED FRUIT | (GF) (DF) (NF) (SF) (NS) (EF) (V) | *Makes 1½ cups*

This flavorful dressing gets its creaminess from tahini, a paste made from raw sesame seeds. Sesame seeds are an excellent source of minerals, including manganese, copper, and calcium, and when compared to other nuts and seeds, they contain the highest amount of phytosterols, which are thought to lower bad cholesterol. When paired with the capsaicin naturally found in jalapeños, this tasty salad dressing may help reduce inflammation and promote healthy blood flow. Depending on how spicy you like your dressing, feel free to include or omit the jalapeño seeds to taste, or start with just half of the jalapeño called for and add more to taste.

½ cup Raw Tahini
(page 180)

¼ cup freshly squeezed
lemon juice

2 cloves garlic, minced

1 jalapeño, minced
(seeds optional)

½ teaspoon sea salt

1 tablespoon extra-virgin
olive oil

½ cup water

Combine all of the ingredients in a blender and blend until completely smooth and creamy. Store in a sealed container in the refrigerator for at least 1 hour before serving, to allow the flavors to develop. Leftovers should keep for up to 1 week when chilled.

NOTE: *Store your salad dressing in sealed glass jars, instead of using plastic containers, to avoid chemicals leaching into your food. Glass Mason jars and leftover jelly or nut butter jars work well and are a great way to reduce waste at the same time.*

honey dijon dressing

NEUTRAL | GF DF NF SF EF | *Makes 1 cup*

An upgrade from traditional honey-mustard dressing, this recipe features a complex blend of ginger, garlic, and honey—an unexpected combination that is shockingly addictive. Consider it a grown-up version of the classic childhood favorite. (Pictured on page 74.)

¼ cup Dijon or stone-ground mustard

2 tablespoons raw apple cider vinegar

¼ cup extra-virgin olive oil

1 clove garlic

1 tablespoon minced fresh ginger (about a 1-inch knob, peeled)

2 tablespoons raw honey

¼ cup water

Combine all of the ingredients in a high-speed blender and blend until the dressing is completely smooth and emulsified. Store in a sealed container in the refrigerator for up to 1 week, and shake well before serving.

make it vegan Replace the honey with maple syrup.

make it sugar-free Replace the honey with stevia, to taste.

CLOCKWISE FROM TOP: Honey Dijon Dressing (page 73), Hemp Seed Ranch (page 76), and Everyday Basil Vinaigrette

everyday basil vinaigrette

NEUTRAL | GF DF NF SF EF | *Makes 1 cup*

This dressing is versatile enough to enjoy over any number of salad combinations, which is why you may find yourself wanting to use it every day. Fresh basil offers a bright taste of summer, but feel free to use any other fresh herb in its place, such as dill or cilantro.

3 tablespoons raw apple cider vinegar

¼ cup fresh basil leaves, tightly packed

6 tablespoons extra-virgin olive oil

2 tablespoons water

2 teaspoons Dijon mustard

2 cloves garlic, minced

2 tablespoons raw honey

Combine all of the ingredients in a blender and blend until completely smooth and emulsified, about 1 minute. Store in a sealed container in the refrigerator for at least 1 hour to allow the flavors to develop, and shake well before serving. Leftovers should keep for up to 1 week when chilled.

NOTE: *Most salad dressings made with olive oil will thicken substantially when chilled in the refrigerator, but adding just a small amount of water to the dressing, as this recipe does, makes it ready to use directly out of the fridge. Feel free to use this trick with any of your other favorite dressing recipes by replacing 2 tablespoons of the olive oil called for with 2 tablespoons of water.*

make it vegan Replace the honey with maple syrup.

make it sugar-free Replace the honey with stevia, to taste.

hemp seed ranch

NUT/SEED/DRIED FRUIT | (GF) (DF) (NF) (SF) (NS) (EF) (V) | *Makes 1½ cups*

This creamy ranch makes a satisfying dip or dressing and packs a punch of protein, thanks to nutrient-rich hemp hearts (see page 26). Using dried herbs, this particular recipe mimics the popular packaged mix and is also just as convenient to prepare. For best results, whip up this dressing the night before you plan on enjoying it, as the flavor gets even better as it sits in the refrigerator. (Pictured on page 74.)

¾ cup water

¼ cup extra-virgin olive oil

1 cup hemp hearts

¾ teaspoon sea salt

1 clove garlic

1 teaspoon Dijon mustard

1 teaspoon onion powder

3 tablespoons freshly
    squeezed lemon juice

2 teaspoons dried chives

1 teaspoon dried parsley

¼ teaspoon dried dill

1. Combine the water, olive oil, hemp hearts, salt, garlic, mustard, onion powder, and lemon juice in a blender and blend until completely smooth and creamy. Scrape down the sides and blend again, if necessary.

2. Add in the dried chives, parsley, and dill and pulse in the blender just enough to combine, but leaving green specks throughout the dressing.

3. This can be served immediately, but for best results store in the refrigerator overnight for the flavor to develop fully. This dressing will thicken when chilled, creating a nice and thick veggie dip, but feel free to thin with additional water, if desired.

NOTE: *Don't use your finger when taste-testing salad dressing, as the flavor will be too concentrated. Instead, use crunchy lettuce, like a romaine leaf, which will more accurately mimic the flavor of the dressing over a large salad.*

go-to greek salad

ANIMAL PROTEIN | (GF) (NF) (SF) (NS) (EF) | *Serves 4*

This classic salad is an easy go-to dish when entertaining a crowd. Crunchy romaine, crisp cucumbers, sweet tomatoes, salty olives, and creamy feta make for a tasty combination of textures and flavors that everyone will love. The smaller you chop these ingredients, the better, ensuring a little bit of everything is included in each forkful.

DRESSING

6 tablespoons extra-virgin olive oil

3 tablespoons freshly squeezed lemon juice

2 cloves garlic

1 teaspoon dried oregano

¼ teaspoon sea salt

¼ teaspoon freshly ground black pepper

SALAD

1 large head romaine lettuce, chopped

1 cucumber, chopped

2 tomatoes, chopped

1 red bell pepper, seeded and chopped

¼ red onion, chopped

½ cup sliced olives

6 ounces raw goat's milk feta, crumbled

1. Prepare the dressing: Combine all of the dressing ingredients in a high-speed blender and blend until completely smooth, making sure the oil is emulsified.

2. Prepare the salad: In a large bowl, combine all of the salad ingredients and pour the dressing over the top. Toss well to coat and serve immediately.

make it vegan Omit the feta, and add sliced avocado instead.

roasted vegetable salad with shallot vinaigrette

STARCH | GF DF NF SF EF V | *Serves 4*

This salad is hearty enough to be served as a meal, thanks to a topping of warm roasted vegetables and creamy avocado. Because fresh artichokes can be tricky to work with, using frozen artichoke hearts will make things easier, without the preservatives found in the canned variety. Tender asparagus spears and meaty artichoke hearts add the perfect texture over crisp romaine lettuce, but feel free to use any other vegetables that may be in season. The result is delicious even when chilled, so you may want to prepare extra roasted vegetables to serve over your salads all week long.

1 pound asparagus spears, cut into 1½-inch pieces

12 ounces frozen artichoke hearts, thawed (about 2½ cups)

3 Roma tomatoes, sliced ½ inch thick

2 tablespoons melted coconut oil

Sea salt

2 heads romaine lettuce, chopped

1 Roasted Red Bell Pepper (page 181), chopped

1 ripe avocado, pitted and chopped

SHALLOT VINAIGRETTE

2 tablespoons raw apple cider vinegar

1 tablespoon finely minced shallot

2 tablespoons maple syrup

⅓ cup extra-virgin olive oil

2 tablespoons water

2 teaspoons Dijon mustard

1 clove garlic, minced

1. Preheat the oven to 350°F and line two rimmed baking sheets with parchment paper.

2. Combine the asparagus, artichoke hearts, and sliced tomatoes in a large bowl and toss with the melted coconut oil. Arrange the vegetables in a single layer on the lined baking sheets, sprinkle with sea salt, and roast in the oven until tender, about 30 minutes. Remove from the oven and allow the vegetables to cool slightly.

3. Prepare the vinaigrette: Combine the vinaigrette ingredients in a high-speed blender and blend until completely smooth. Set aside.

4. Place the chopped romaine in a large serving bowl and top with the warm roasted vegetables, roasted pepper, and chopped avocado. Pour the dressing over the top and toss well to coat. Serve immediately.

make it omnivore-friendly Omit the avocado and add a serving of high-quality cooked meat, fish, or goat cheese on top of this salad instead.

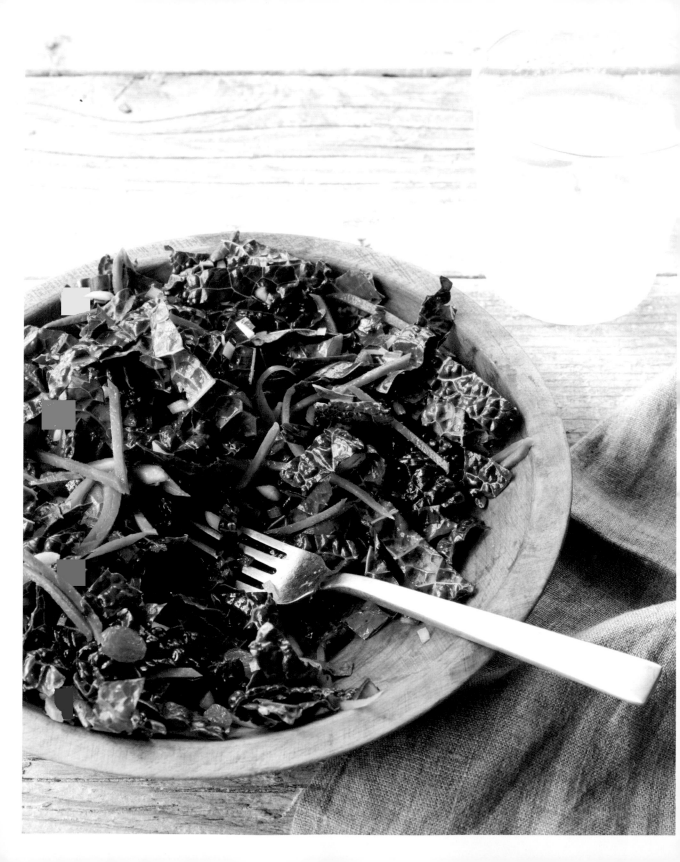

creamy caesar salad

NUT/SEED/DRIED FRUIT | GF DF SF NS EF V | *Serves 4*

This classic salad is a favorite in restaurants, but it isn't so healthy when smothered in cheese and croutons. Instead, this raw and vegan dressing gets its creaminess from cashews, which contain less fat than most other nuts and are packed with heart-healthy antioxidants and minerals like copper, magnesium, and zinc. Garlic provides this dressing with its signature flavor, along with a multitude of health benefits, but beware of its lingering aftertaste—you may not want to serve this salad on a first date!

DRESSING

¾ cup water

1 cup raw whole cashews, soaked for 2 hours and rinsed well (see page 28)

1 teaspoon Dijon mustard

5 cloves garlic

¼ cup freshly squeezed lemon juice

1 teaspoon raw apple cider vinegar

2 tablespoons extra-virgin olive oil

1 teaspoon sea salt

2 heads romaine, chopped

Walnut "Parmesan," for topping (optional; page 181)

1. Prepare the dressing: Combine all of the dressing ingredients in a high-speed blender and blend until completely smooth and creamy.

2. Pour a generous amount of dressing over the chopped romaine and toss well to coat. Serve with a sprinkling of Walnut "Parmesan" on top. Leftover dressing can be stored in a sealed container in the refrigerator for up to 3 days.

chinese cabbage salad

NEUTRAL | GF DF SF EF | *Serves 4*

This salad was inspired by one of my favorite restaurants in Los Angeles, which serves an addictive Chinese chicken salad. An explosion of flavors and textures keeps each bite unique and utterly irresistible. What I love about this marinated salad is that it can be made ahead of time and actually tastes better the next day. Try bringing it to your next potluck and enjoy the leftovers as an easily packed lunch during the week.

DRESSING

¼ cup coconut vinegar

⅓ cup extra-virgin olive oil

1 teaspoon minced ginger

1 teaspoon minced garlic

3 tablespoons raw honey

½ teaspoon toasted
   sesame oil

SALAD

8 cups shredded cabbage

2 carrots, shredded

½ red onion, chopped

Chopped fresh cilantro,
   for garnish

TOPPINGS (OPTIONAL)

Slivered raw almonds
   or sunflower seeds (NUT/
   SEED/DRIED FRUIT) or
   sliced avocado (STARCH)

1. Prepare the dressing: Combine all of the dressing ingredients in a high-powered blender and blend until completely smooth.

2. Prepare the salad: Combine the shredded cabbage, carrots, and onion in a large bowl and pour the dressing over the top. Toss well to coat and let marinate in the refrigerator for at least 1 hour.

3. Garnish with fresh chopped cilantro right before serving, and use one of the toppings.

make it vegan Replace the honey with maple syrup.

make it sugar-free Replace the honey with stevia, to taste.

make it omnivore-friendly Skip the additional toppings and add your favorite high-quality meat to this dish.

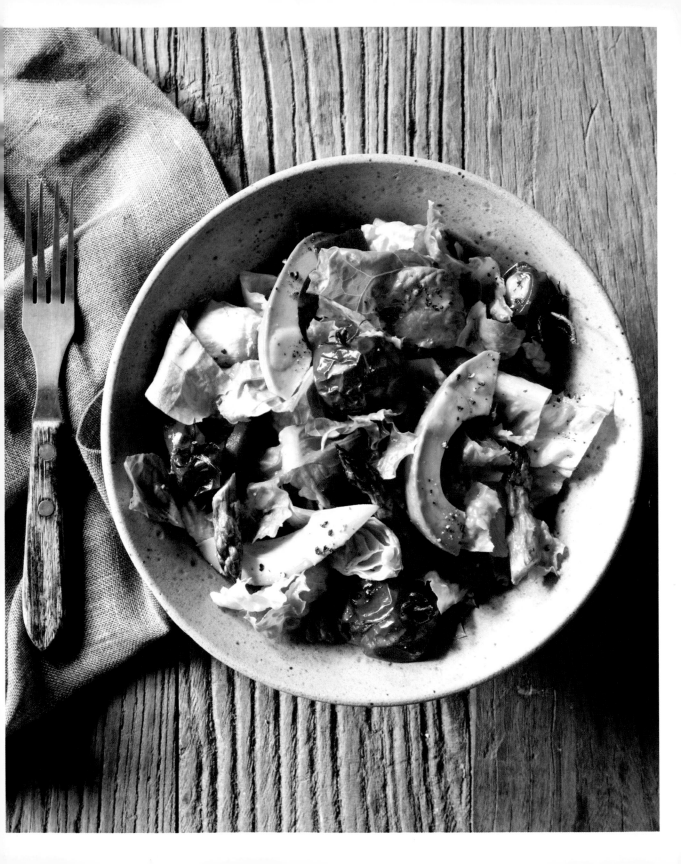

no-fail kale salad

NUT/SEED/DRIED FRUIT | GF DF SF EF | *Serves 4*

Kale's chewy and fibrous leaves can make it a bit daunting, but when paired with a lemony dressing, along with sweet and crunchy toppings, it is transformed into a delectable dish. The key to a perfect kale salad is to finely chop the leaves so the pieces are small enough to pick up a little bit of everything in each bite. Next, you must get your hands dirty—literally—by massaging the dressing into the leaves, making them more tender and easier to digest. The end result is a beautifully composed salad, loaded with calcium, iron, and vitamins A, C, and K, that is bursting with flavor in each bite.

LEMON DRESSING
¼ cup freshly squeezed lemon juice
¼ cup extra-virgin olive oil
2 tablespoons raw honey
1 clove garlic, minced
¼ teaspoon sea salt

1 pound kale leaves, stems removed (about 2 bunches)
¼ red onion, diced
2 carrots, shredded
½ cup golden raisins
½ cup slivered almonds

1. Prepare the dressing: Combine all of the dressing ingredients in a small jar with a lid; shake vigorously to mix. Set aside.

2. Use a sharp knife to chop the kale leaves into small pieces—the smaller, the better. Place the chopped leaves in a large bowl and add the red onion and shredded carrots.

3. Pour the dressing over the vegetables and use your hands to massage the salad. After just a few minutes of squeezing the leaves between your hands, they will turn a darker green and have a wilted, silky texture, similar to that of cooked kale.

4. Add the raisins and almonds and toss well to mix. Store in the refrigerator until ready to serve or serve immediately.

NOTE: *This salad is sturdy enough to store in the refrigerator for up to 3 days, even with the dressing mixed in.*

make it vegan Replace the honey with maple syrup.

mediterranean chopped salad

NEUTRAL | (GF) (NF) (SF) (NS) (EF) | *Serves 4 to 6*

This chopped salad is the perfect make-ahead dish, calling for firm vegetables that won't get soggy the way tender leafy greens do. In fact, the flavor of this summery salad actually gets better the longer it marinates in the refrigerator, so feel free to make it several hours, or even a day, in advance and enjoy it as an easy pre-dinner salad or packed lunch. I love to add crumbled feta to this dish for extra Mediterranean flair, but it can be left out for a vegan-friendly and dairy-free dish. In fact, this salad is completely customizable to suit your tastes and dietary needs, so get creative with the toppings and use any seasonal produce that you have on hand.

3 tablespoons freshly
squeezed lemon juice

2 tablespoons extra-virgin
olive oil

1 clove garlic, minced

¼ teaspoon sea salt

2 cups chopped tomatoes

2 cups chopped cucumber

½ red onion, chopped

1 red bell pepper, seeded
and chopped

½ cup pitted and chopped
olives

½ cup fresh chopped
parsley

½ cup fresh chopped dill

Freshly ground black
pepper

TOPPINGS (OPTIONAL)

6 ounces crumbled raw
goat's milk feta (ANIMAL
PROTEIN) or 1 avocado,
pitted and sliced (STARCH)

1. In a large bowl, whisk together the lemon juice, olive oil, garlic, and salt. Add the tomatoes, cucumber, onion, bell pepper, olives, parsley, and dill and mix well. Season with pepper and additional sea salt, if desired.

2. Let the salad stand at room temperature for 20 minutes to blend the flavors, then top with crumbled feta or sliced avocado right before serving. Store leftovers in the refrigerator for up to 3 days. For best results, let the salad come to room temperature again before serving.

quinoa tabouli

STARCH | (GF) (DF) (NF) (SF) (NS) (EF) (V) | *Serves 4 to 6*

This Middle Eastern salad dish is as refreshing as it gets, starring garden-fresh parsley and cooling mint. Combined with protein-rich quinoa, sweet tomatoes, and hydrating cucumber, this tabouli makes for a filling meal that won't weigh you down.

1 cup quinoa, rinsed and drained

2 cups water

3 tablespoons freshly squeezed lemon juice

¼ cup extra-virgin olive oil

1 clove garlic, minced

1 teaspoon salt

1 cup flat-leaf parsley, chopped

¼ cup chopped fresh mint leaves

2 green onions, white and green parts, chopped

2 cups chopped tomatoes

2 cups diced cucumber

1. In a small saucepan, add the quinoa and water and bring to a boil. Cover and lower the heat, cooking until all of the water is absorbed and the quinoa is tender, about 15 minutes. Allow the quinoa to cool. (Place it in the refrigerator to speed the cooling process.)

2. In a large bowl, whisk together the fresh lemon juice, olive oil, garlic, and salt. Add the parsley, mint, onions, tomatoes, and cucumber and toss well to coat.

3. Add in the cooled quinoa, and stir well to combine. Serve immediately or store in the refrigerator for up to 3 days.

almond pulp hummus

NUT/SEED/DRIED FRUIT | (GF) (DF) (SF) (NS) (EF) (V) | *Serves 4 to 6*

When you start making your own almond milk, you may find yourself with quite a bit of leftover almond pulp on your hands. This pulp can be dried and made into flour, but the process is time-consuming and the resulting flour doesn't always work well in recipes. Instead, this hummus calls for the wet pulp left over from making almond milk, so there's no extra drying process involved. The resulting hummus has an extra dose of fiber and is easier to digest without the chickpeas found in traditional recipes. Serve with raw vegetables of your choice or Crispy Zucchini Chips (page 95).

⅓ cup Raw Tahini (page 180)

¼ cup freshly squeezed lemon juice

1 tablespoon ground cumin

2 cloves garlic, minced

½ teaspoon sea salt

¼ cup extra-virgin olive oil

1 scant cup wet almond pulp, left over from making 1 batch of Homemade Almond Milk (page 178)

¼ cup water

1. Combine the tahini, lemon juice, cumin, garlic, salt, and olive oil in a high-speed blender and blend until smooth.

2. Add the almond pulp and water, then blend again until very smooth. For best flavor, place the hummus in the refrigerator for 2 hours before serving. Store in a sealed container in the refrigerator for up to 1 week.

NOTE: *A high-speed blender is best for breaking down the gritty texture of the almond pulp, but a food processor can also be used to prepare this hummus.*

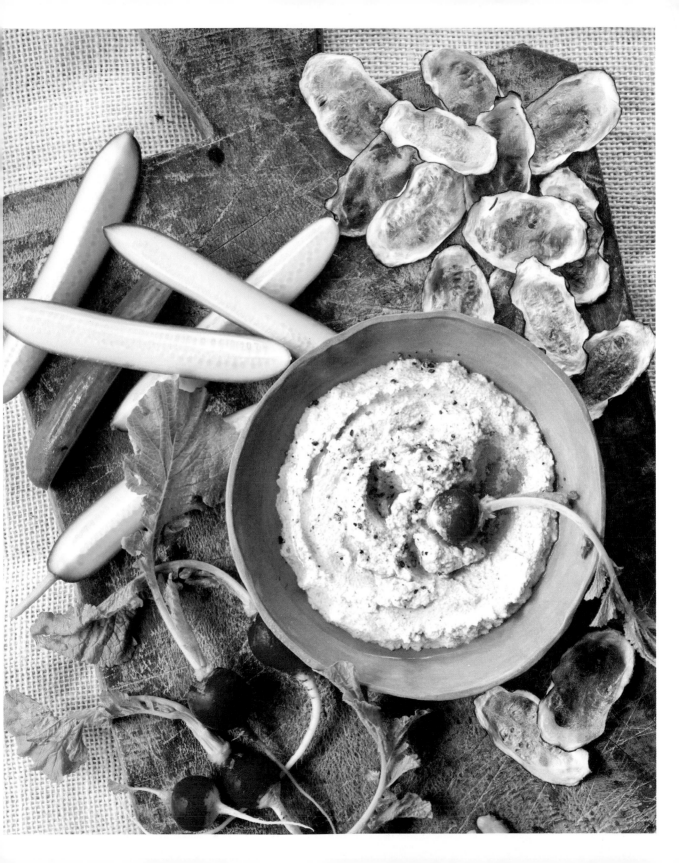

spinach artichoke dip

NEUTRAL | GF DF NF SF NS EF V | *Makes 3 cups*

This thick and flavorful dip is loaded with antioxidants, without the need for cheese or additional thickeners. Fresh artichokes can be intimidating to work with, but frozen artichoke hearts are easily thawed overnight in the refrigerator and are ready to use directly from the bag, without the preservatives often found in the canned variety. Paired with spinach and roasted red bell pepper, plus a little nutritional yeast for a "cheesy" flavor, this dip is a lighter and healthier alternative that you can enjoy with your favorite chips or raw crudités.

10 ounces frozen spinach, thawed and drained

12 ounces frozen artichoke hearts, thawed

1 Roasted Red Bell Pepper (page 181), chopped

1 clove garlic, minced

¼ cup diced red onion

2 tablespoons freshly squeezed lemon juice

¼ cup extra-virgin olive oil

¼ cup nutritional yeast (optional)

1½ teaspoons sea salt

In a large food processor fitted with the "S" blade, combine all of the ingredients and process until a relatively smooth dip is created. Adjust the seasoning to taste and transfer to a sealed container to chill in the refrigerator for at least 2 hours before serving, to allow the flavors to meld. Serve chilled and store leftovers in the refrigerator for up to 3 days.

NOTE: *This dip also makes a delicious pasta sauce. Simply toss it with your favorite freshly cooked pasta for a warm weeknight meal or store it in the refrigerator for an easy chilled pasta salad.*

simple sautéed kale

NEUTRAL | GF DF NF SF NS EF V | *Serves 4*

This dish is just about as simple as it gets, but with these fresh and flavorful ingredients, less is more. Cooked kale has a tender, almost silky, texture, and when paired with garlic, salt, and coconut oil, it becomes downright delectable. Don't be overwhelmed by the large quantity of raw kale this recipe calls for, as it will shrink significantly when cooked.

1 tablespoon coconut oil

4 cloves garlic, minced

1 pound curly kale, stems removed and coarsely chopped (2 bunches)

¼ cup water

Sea salt

1. Melt the coconut oil in a large stockpot or enameled Dutch oven over medium heat. Add the garlic and sauté until fragrant, about 1 minute.

2. Add the chopped kale and water and toss to coat. Cover and cook for 5 minutes. Remove the lid and stir well, cooking until all of the liquid has evaporated. Season generously with salt and serve warm.

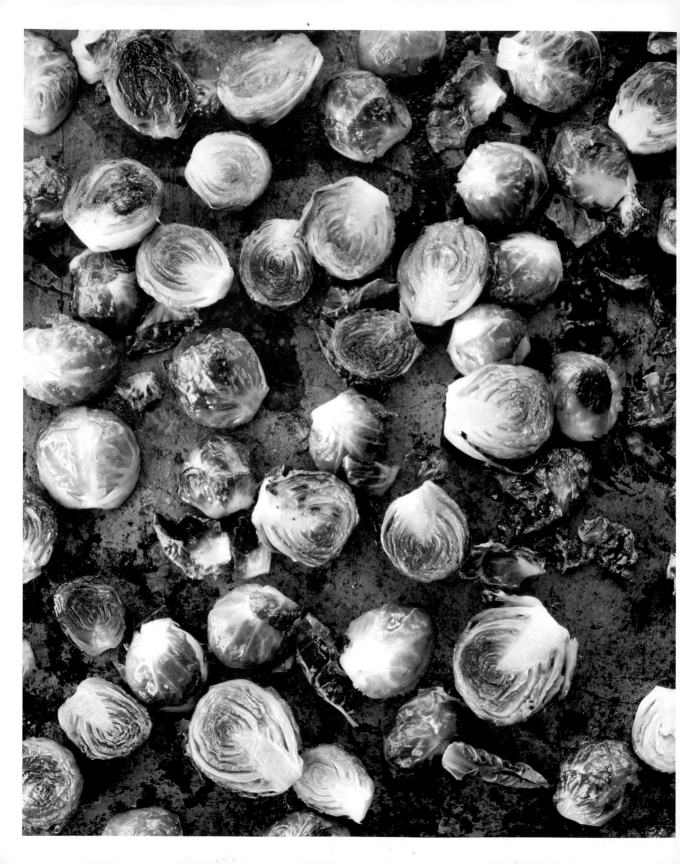

salt & vinegar brussels sprouts

NEUTRAL | (GF) (DF) (NF) (SF) (NS) (EF) (V) | *Serves 4*

These roasted brussels sprouts are my solution to any salty craving. They are just as addictive as French fries, but unlike those greasy spuds, they digest seamlessly with any meal and don't require a deep-fryer. Though brussels sprouts aren't typically a favorite among non-veggie lovers, I urge you to give these tender green buds a chance—you may be surprised to hear your family begging for more!

2 tablespoons melted coconut oil

1 tablespoon raw apple cider vinegar

½ teaspoon sea salt

1 pound brussels sprouts, halved

1. Preheat the oven to 350°F.

2. In a large bowl, stir together the melted coconut oil, vinegar, and salt, then add the sliced brussels sprouts and toss well to coat. (Don't be afraid to get your hands dirty—rub the mixture into the sprouts well!)

3. Arrange the coated brussels sprouts in a single layer on a baking sheet, cut side down, and roast them until golden and tender, 25 to 30 minutes. Serve immediately.

seasoned sweet potato home fries

STARCH | (GF) (DF) (NF) (SF) (NS) (EF) (V) | *Serves 4 to 6*

These home fries are a comforting side dish, with a sweet, spicy, and salty flavor that's hard to resist. Because these spuds are baked, not fried, they are a healthier alternative to French fries and supply a healthy amount of fiber, potassium, and vitamin A in each serving. A coating of dried herbs helps these potatoes crisp up, but feel free to use any spices you like—the possibilities are endless. For the greatest nutrition content, don't peel your potatoes, as this is where most of their nutrients lie. (Pictured on page 111.)

2 pounds sweet potatoes, cut into 1-inch chunks or wedges

2 tablespoons melted coconut oil

1 teaspoon ground paprika

1 teaspoon garlic powder

1 teaspoon onion powder

1 teaspoon sea salt

1. Preheat the oven to 350°F.

2. In a large bowl, toss the sweet potato chunks with the melted coconut oil. Sprinkle the paprika, garlic powder, onion powder, and sea salt over the potatoes and toss again to coat evenly.

3. Arrange the potatoes in a single layer on two rimmed baking sheets and bake for 20 minutes. Flip the potatoes for even browning, then return to the oven to bake until the edges of the potatoes start to brown, about 20 minutes more. Serve immediately.

cheesy garlic & herb cauliflower mash

ANIMAL PROTEIN | (GF) (NF) (SF) (NS) (EF) | *Serves 4 to 6*

Mashed cauliflower is a lighter alternative to starchy white potatoes and is particularly satisfying when combined with aromatic garlic and herbs. The addition of soft goat cheese makes these "faux-tatoes" extra fluffy and creamy, while still being properly combined for a classic meat-and-potatoes-style dinner. For a dairy-free version, leave out the cheese, creating a neutral side dish that will digest easily with any meal.

1 tablespoon butter or coconut oil

4 cloves garlic, minced

½ cup water

1 (2½-pound) head cauliflower, cut into florets

2 teaspoons minced fresh thyme leaves

2 teaspoons minced fresh sage leaves

¼ cup chèvre (soft goat cheese)

1 to 2 teaspoons sea salt

Freshly ground black pepper

1. Melt the butter in a large stockpot or enameled Dutch oven over medium heat. Add the garlic and sauté until fragrant, about 1 minute. Add the water and the cauliflower florets, and bring to a boil. Cover and lower the heat, steaming until the cauliflower is easily pierced with a fork, about 15 minutes.

2. Transfer the cooked garlic and cauliflower, along with any remaining liquid in the pot, to a large food processor fitted with an "S" blade. Add the thyme, sage, and chèvre and season with salt and pepper to taste. Process until the cauliflower is pureed, with a fluffy texture similar to that of mashed potatoes.

3. Adjust any seasonings to taste, then return the mixture to medium heat. Stir well to heat throughout, then serve warm.

make it vegan Use coconut oil instead of butter and omit the goat cheese. The result will be slightly less creamy but just as flavorful with an extra pinch of salt.

classic guacamole

STARCH OR FRESH FRUIT | GF DF NF SF NS EF V | *Serves 4 to 6*

Guacamole is a naturally detox-friendly dip, featuring fiber-rich avocados and freshly squeezed lemon juice. It can be whipped together in minutes, using any ingredients you like, but this recipe is my go-to formula for creating a flawless flavor every time. For best results, be sure to use ripe avocados that give slightly when pressed with your fingers.

3 ripe avocados, pitted

1 tomato, chopped and seeded

¼ sweet white onion, diced

1 clove garlic, minced

2 tablespoons finely diced jalapeño

2 tablespoons fresh chopped cilantro

1 to 3 tablespoons freshly squeezed lemon juice, as desired for tartness

Sea salt and black pepper

1. Scoop the flesh of the avocados into a large bowl and mash with a fork, leaving the texture slightly chunky.

2. Add in the tomato, onion, garlic, jalapeño, cilantro, and 1 tablespoon of the lemon juice, then season with salt and pepper. Stir well and taste the mixture, and then continue to add the lemon juice 1 tablespoon at a time until the desired tartness has been reached. Enjoy immediately or set aside for up to 1 hour before serving for the flavors to fully develop.

NOTE: *I like to use a Microplane to quickly grate a clove of raw garlic into a dish like this one. It's faster than mincing the garlic with a knife, and it grates the garlic into a finer consistency, so the flavor is evenly distributed throughout the whole dip.*

crispy zucchini chips

NEUTRAL | (GF) (DF) (NF) (SF) (NS) (EF) (V) | *Serves 2*

These zucchini chips are the closest I've come to satisfying a crunchy, salty craving, without all of the starch or deep-frying of regular potato chips. The key to creating these crispy chips is cutting the zucchini ultrathin, then baking the slices at a low temperature to avoid burning. For best results, use a mandoline, which will quickly and easily create uniform zucchini slices, and be sure to use a light touch when salting, as these chips will shrink when baked, concentrating their salty flavor. Though this recipe creates two trays of zucchini chips, I recommend doubling the batch if you plan on serving more than two people—they will disappear quickly! (Pictured on page 87.)

1 large zucchini

2 teaspoons melted coconut oil

Sea salt

1. Preheat the oven to 250°F and line two rimmed baking sheets with parchment paper.

2. Use a mandoline or sharp knife to cut the zucchini, on a diagonal, into slices $\frac{1}{16}$ inch thick. The thinner the slices, the crispier the chips will be.

3. In a large bowl, toss the sliced zucchini with the melted coconut oil, using your hands to make sure each slice is lightly coated.

4. Arrange the zucchini slices in a single layer on each baking sheet, making sure that each slice is flat against the baking sheet without overlapping. Sprinkle lightly with sea salt and bake for 40 minutes.

5. Open the oven door to see if the slices are starting to brown and remove any slices that are already crisp, to avoid burning. Flip the remaining slices, then return them to the oven and continue baking, checking every 5 minutes, until all of the slices are golden and crisp. Let the chips cool before serving.

NOTE: *Cutting the zucchini on a diagonal creates slightly larger slices, which is helpful because these slices will shrink when baked. For a colorful variety of veggie chips, try using this method to create chips out of carrots, parsnips, or beets, too.*

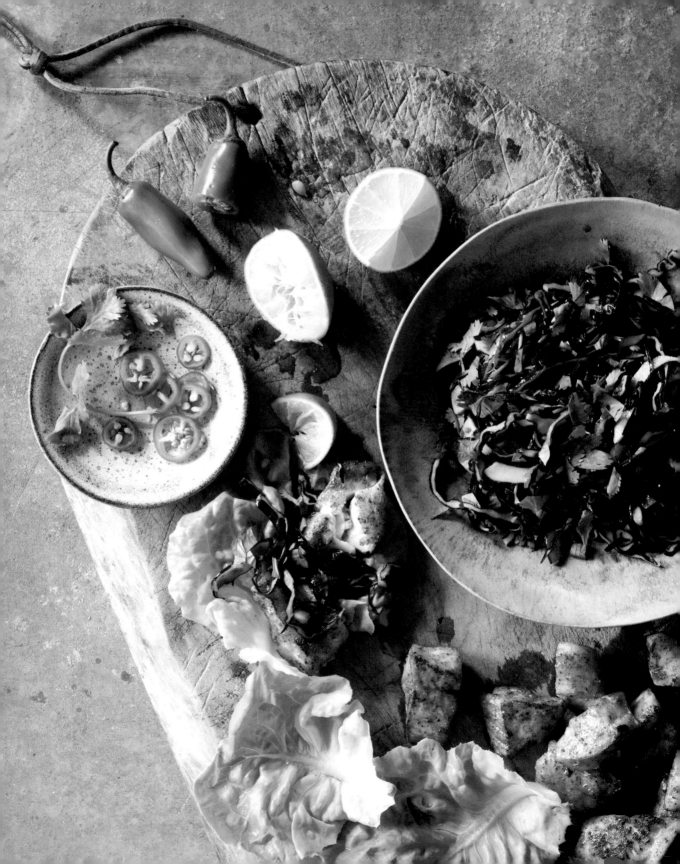

soups, sandwiches & wraps

Though they are often ordered with good intentions, many soups, sandwiches, and wraps at your local deli are loaded with refined flour, sugar, and fillers, making them nutritionally lacking and difficult to digest. Instead, the following recipes are ultracomforting and jam-packed with nutrition, without sacrificing the tastes or textures you love. For a light, yet filling meal, try the flavorful Raw Falafel Wraps (page 106) loaded with your favorite veggies, or warm up with a hearty bowl of Lentil Chili (page 104) or creamy Broccoli Cheese Soup (page 101). Vegetables have never tasted so good!

carrot ginger soup

NEUTRAL | **GF** **DF** **SF** **NF** **NS** **EF** **V** | *Serves 4*

This velvety carrot soup will warm you inside and out, thanks to the addition of freshly minced ginger. You'll be amazed at how creamy this soup becomes, even without the use of heavy cream. This recipe packs a hefty dose of spicy ginger, but if you'd prefer a more mild-tasting soup, feel free to start with just half the amount and add more to your taste.

1 teaspoon coconut oil

1 yellow onion, chopped

2 cloves garlic, minced

1 pound carrots, chopped (about 3 cups)

3 cups water

1½ teaspoons sea salt

2 tablespoons freshly minced ginger

½ cup coconut milk (see note)

1. Melt the coconut oil in a large stockpot over medium heat and sauté the onion until tender, 8 to 10 minutes. Add the garlic and sauté until fragrant, about 1 minute.

2. Add the carrots, water, salt, and ginger, then bring to a boil. Lower the heat to a simmer, then cover and cook until the carrots are easily pierced with a fork, about 20 minutes.

3. Transfer the soup to a blender or food processor and process until smooth. (When blending hot liquids, be sure to remove the plastic cap from the blender lid and cover the opening with a dish towel to allow steam to escape and prevent burns.) Alternatively, you could use an immersion blender directly in the stockpot.

4. Return the soup to the stockpot over medium heat, stir in the coconut milk, and heat to the desired serving temperature. Serve immediately.

NOTE: *You can use Fresh Coconut Milk (page 175) or canned coconut milk in this recipe, both with excellent results. When using canned coconut milk, look for cans that are labeled BPA-free.*

red bell pepper & tomato bisque

NEUTRAL | GF DF SF NS EF V | *Serves 4 to 6*

Classic tomato gets an upgrade in this slightly sweet and savory soup, thanks to the addition of a naturally sweet roasted red bell pepper. Even without the use of heavy cream, this soup becomes smooth and creamy when blended in a high-speed blender. Round it out with a splash of almond milk for a dairy-free finish.

1 teaspoon coconut oil or butter

2 large carrots, chopped

1 yellow onion, chopped

1 (28-ounce) box or jar chopped tomatoes

1 cup water

2 cloves garlic, minced

1 tablespoon dried basil

1½ teaspoons sea salt

1 Roasted Red Bell Pepper, chopped (page 181)

1 cup Homemade Almond Milk (page 178; see note)

1. Melt the coconut oil in a large stockpot over medium heat and sauté the carrots and onion until tender, about 10 minutes.

2. Add the tomatoes, water, garlic, basil, salt, and bell pepper and bring the soup to a boil. Lower the heat and cover, simmering for 30 to 45 minutes, until the vegetables are very tender.

3. Transfer the soup in batches to a high-speed blender and blend until very smooth. (When blending hot liquids, be sure to remove the plastic cap from the blender lid and cover the opening with a dish towel to allow steam to escape and prevent burns.)

4. Return to medium heat, stir in the almond milk, and heat thoroughly. Adjust the seasoning to taste, if necessary, and serve warm.

NOTE: *Store-bought almond milk often contains preservatives that give it an undesirable flavor. If homemade almond milk is not an option, replace it with pure water.*

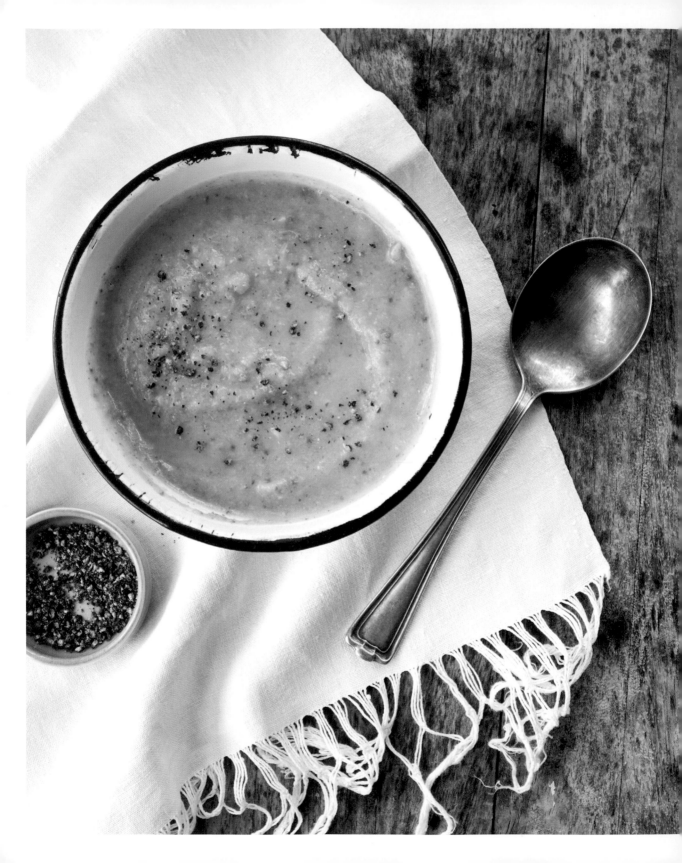

broccoli cheese soup

ANIMAL PROTEIN | (GF) (NF) (SF) (NS) (EF) | *Serves 4 to 6*

This creamy soup has all of the comfort of traditional Cheddar broccoli soup, with just a fraction of the cheese and without the need for flour or additional thickeners. Broccoli is bursting with vitamin C, and just one serving of this soup provides 100 percent of your recommended daily intake, and it also contains a compound called sulforaphane, which could help fight osteoarthritis, the most common form of arthritis.[1] Blended with aromatic vegetables, this soup is sure to have your whole family enjoying their veggies.

1 teaspoon butter or
  coconut oil
½ yellow onion, chopped
2 carrots, chopped
2 celery stalks, chopped
2 cloves garlic, minced
1 pound broccoli florets
3½ cups water
¼ cup chèvre
  (soft goat cheese)
Sea salt and freshly
  ground black pepper
Ground nutmeg, for
  garnish (optional)

1. Melt the butter in a large stockpot over medium heat and sauté the onion, carrots, and celery until tender, about 8 minutes. Add the garlic and sauté for another minute, just until fragrant.

2. Add the broccoli and water and bring the soup to a boil. Cover, lower the heat, and simmer for 30 minutes, or until the vegetables are very tender, then stir in the chèvre and 1 teaspoon of sea salt.

3. Use an immersion blender to blend the soup directly in the pot. Depending on your desired texture, you can leave it slightly chunky or make it silky smooth. (Alternatively, you can use a blender or food processor, but you may need to blend the soup in batches.) Season with pepper and additional salt to taste, then serve warm with a pinch of ground nutmeg on top.

curried sweet potato bisque

STARCH | GF DF SF NS EF V | *Serves 4 to 6*

This sweet and spicy soup has become a staple in our home when the weather cools down. It's filling enough to be enjoyed as a meal but also makes a delicious addition to any lunch or dinner. When preparing soups, I prefer to use water in lieu of vegetable stock, as it saves both time and money. Cooking the vegetables and seasonings in water still provides plenty of flavor, without the additional step of preparing and storing a homemade stock or purchasing a boxed version.

1 teaspoon coconut oil

1 yellow onion, chopped

2 cloves garlic, minced

2 pounds sweet potatoes, peeled and chopped

2 teaspoons curry powder

1½ teaspoons sea salt

3 cups water

½ cup Homemade Almond Milk (page 178)

1. Melt the coconut oil in a large stockpot over medium heat and sauté the onion and garlic until very soft, about 10 minutes.

2. Add the sweet potatoes, curry powder, salt, and water and bring to a boil. Lower the heat to a simmer, then cover and cook until the sweet potatoes are fork-tender, about 15 minutes.

3. Use an immersion blender to blend the soup directly in the pot, or carefully transfer the soup, in batches, to a food processor or blender, and then carefully blend into a silky-smooth consistency. (When blending hot liquids, be sure to remove the plastic cap from the blender lid, and cover the opening with a dish towel to allow steam to escape and to prevent burns.)

4. Return the blended soup to the stockpot, stir in the almond milk, then heat and serve warm.

creamy asparagus soup

NEUTRAL | (GF) (DF) (NF) (SF) (NS) (EF) (V) | *Serves 4 to 6*

This delicate soup pairs well with any meal and is an excellent way to enjoy the nutritional benefits of asparagus. Loaded with nutrients, this green veggie is a good source of fiber, folate, and vitamins A, C, E, and K and is notably rich in a detoxifying compound called glutathione, which may help protect against certain forms of cancer. So that no one will miss the addition of heavy cream, be sure to blend this soup long enough to achieve a smooth, velvety texture.

1 tablespoon coconut oil

1 yellow onion, chopped

5 cloves garlic, minced

2 pounds fresh asparagus, woody ends discarded, chopped into 1-inch pieces

2 teaspoons sea salt

3 cups water

Freshly ground black pepper, for garnish

Chopped green onions, green parts only, for garnish

1. Melt the coconut oil in a stockpot or enameled Dutch oven over medium heat. Add the onion and garlic and sauté until tender, about 8 minutes. Add the asparagus, salt, and water. Bring the soup to a boil, then cover and lower the heat to a simmer. Simmer until the asparagus is fork-tender, about 20 minutes.

2. Transfer the soup in small batches to a high-speed blender and carefully purée the soup until very smooth, covering the vent at the top of the blender with a dish towel to let steam escape.

3. Return the soup to the stove over medium heat and cook until the desired serving temperature is reached. Serve warm, with a sprinkle of pepper and chopped green onions.

lentil chili

STARCH | **GF** **DF** **NF** **SF** **NS** **EF** **V** | *Serves 4 to 6*

This vegetarian chili makes a great alternative to the traditional meat-based version, as it is loaded with protein, along with an extra boost of filling fiber. Lentils tend to be easier to digest than beans, and because they don't require soaking before they're cooked, they are also a faster and more convenient option for this hearty stew. I like to use red lentils in this recipe for their appealing color and quick cooking time, but feel free to use any other type of lentil that is easily available to you.

1 teaspoon coconut oil

1 yellow onion

3 carrots, chopped

3 celery stalks, chopped

1 red bell pepper, chopped

4 cloves garlic, minced

1 (28-ounce) box or jar
   diced tomatoes

1 cup dry red lentils

1 teaspoon cumin

1 teaspoon chili powder

2 teaspoons sea salt

2 ½ cups water

Chopped parsley,
   for garnish

1. Melt the coconut oil in a large stockpot or enameled Dutch oven over medium heat. Add the onion, carrots, celery, and bell pepper and sauté until tender, about 10 minutes.

2. Add the garlic and sauté just until fragrant, about 1 minute. Add the tomatoes, lentils, cumin, chili powder, salt, and water and bring to a boil. Lower the heat, cover, and let the chili simmer until the lentils are tender, about 30 minutes. Adjust the seasonings to taste and serve warm, garnished with the parsley.

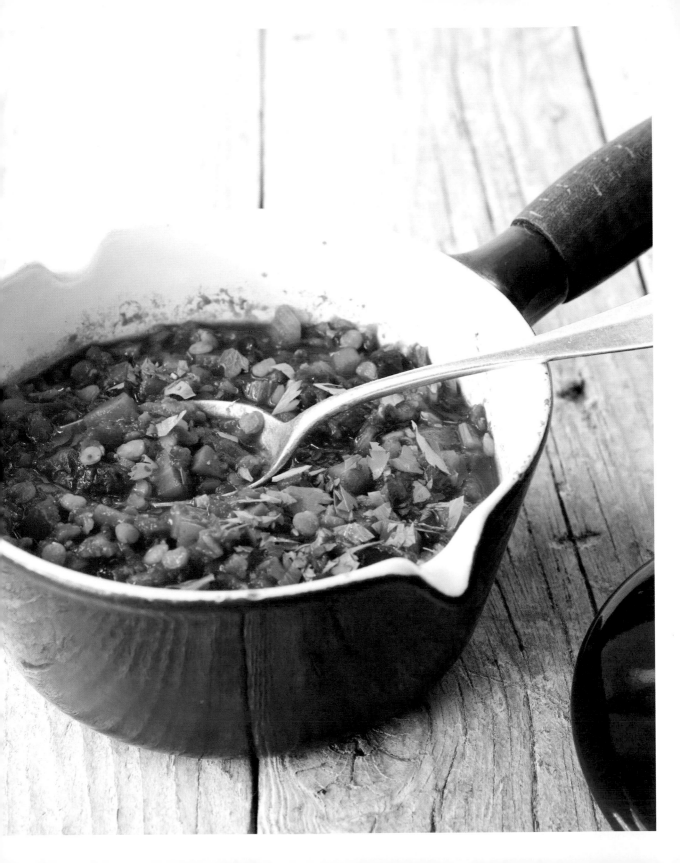

raw falafel wraps

NUT/SEED/DRIED FRUIT | (GF) (DF) (SF) (NS) (EF) (V) | *Serves 4*

A popular Middle Eastern fast food, falafel is typically made from ground chickpeas and then deep-fried and served in a pita. This recipe features the same flavor, but skips the deep-frying process, for a healthier no-bake filling that's even faster to prepare. Just ¼ cup of walnuts fulfills our daily require-ment for omega-3 fatty acids, and these healthy nuts may also help lower cholesterol and reduce inflammation in the body. Because nuts can be difficult to digest when eaten in large quantities, this recipe has been lightened up with the addition of fresh carrots, creating a more hydrating falafel filling that can easily be scooped into a lettuce wrap for an easy packed lunch or afternoon snack.

1 cup raw walnut halves

1 cup diced carrot

2 tablespoons diced red onion

1 teaspoon ground cumin

1 teaspoon ground coriander

¼ cup fresh chopped parsley

¼ cup fresh chopped cilantro

½ teaspoon sea salt

2 tablespoons freshly squeezed lemon juice

2 tablespoons Raw Almond Butter (page 179)

4 to 6 collard leaves, stems removed, for serving

Red bell pepper slices, for serving

Cucumber slices, for serving

1. In a large food processor fitted with an "S" blade, combine the walnuts, carrots, onion, cumin, coriander, parsley, cilantro, and salt. Process for 5 to 10 seconds, until a crumbly mixture is created. Add the lemon juice and almond butter and process again, just until the mixture sticks together.

2. Scoop 2 to 3 tablespoons of the falafel filling into each collard leaf, top with several red bell pepper and cucumber slices, then roll up and devour. Store any leftover filling in an airtight container in the refrigerator for up to 3 days.

NOTE: *The best part about working with raw food is that you can keep tweaking the recipe until it tastes exactly the way you want it to. If you want a spicier falafel filling, add more cumin and coriander, or for a tangier result, add more lemon juice. You can keep adding and adjusting ingredients until the taste is "just right," so you'll never wind up with a recipe flop!*

thai-style lettuce wraps

NUT/SEED/DRIED FRUIT | (GF) (DF) (EF) | *Serves 4 to 6*

Almost completely vegetable-based and free of harmful additives, like MSG, these lettuce wraps are reminiscent of the version served at your favorite Thai-style restaurant. Crunchy pecans provide a meaty texture to this simple filling, but they are added at the end of the cooking process, so as to not damage their delicate oils with high heat. Serve in butter lettuce for a velvety-smooth wrap that is durable enough to hold this warm, delectable filling.

SAUCE

¼ cup tamari

3 tablespoons honey

2 teaspoons raw apple cider vinegar

1 teaspoon minced fresh ginger

1 teaspoon minced garlic

FILLING

2 cups diced carrot

1 cup diced celery

½ yellow onion, diced

1 cup raw pecan halves, briefly pulsed in a food processor

1 head butter lettuce, for serving

1. Prepare the sauce: In a small bowl, whisk together the tamari, honey, vinegar, ginger, and garlic until well mixed.

2. Prepare the filling: In a large saucepan over medium heat, combine the carrot, celery, and onion and cover with the sauce. Bring the sauce to a simmer, then cover and allow the vegetables to cook until fork-tender, 10 to 15 minutes.

3. Remove the lid and increase the heat, bringing the sauce to a boil. Allow the sauce to boil until the liquid evaporates, then remove from the heat. Add the pulsed pecan pieces and stir well to coat. Let the mixture marinate for 5 minutes, then scoop into butter lettuce leaves and serve.

make it **vegan** Replace the honey with maple syrup.

make it **sugar-free** Replace the honey with stevia, to taste.

make it **soy-free** Replace the tamari with coconut aminos.

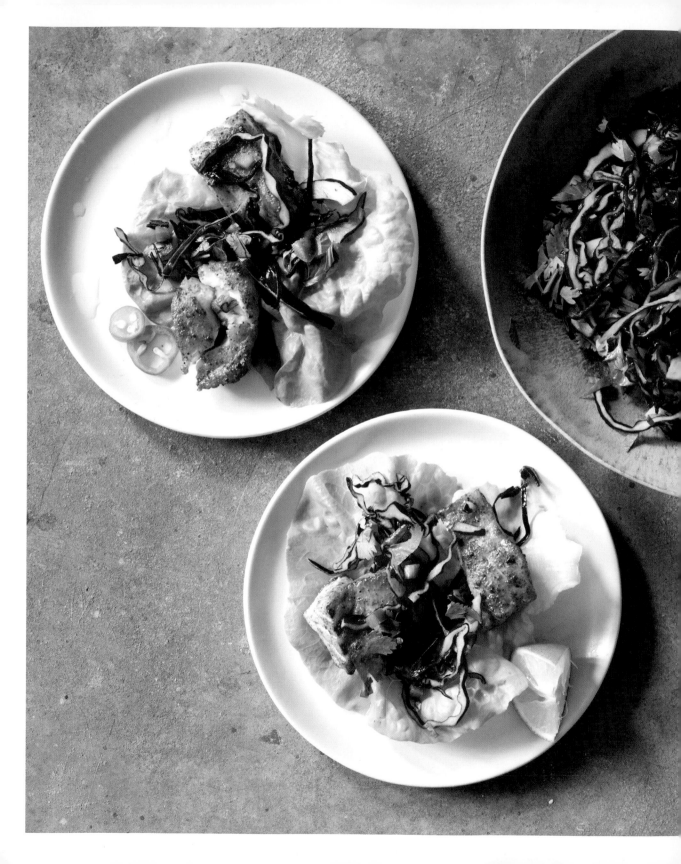

skillet fish tacos with citrus slaw

ANIMAL PROTEIN | GF DF NF SF EF | *Serves 4*

These fish tacos are a refreshing change of pace from the traditional meat and cheese variety and are also lighter on your digestion. Paired with a bright slaw and served in velvety butter lettuce, these tacos are loaded with live enzymes, omega-3 fatty acids, and vitamin K, which help keep your mind sharp. Wild-caught cod works well in this recipe, but any other mild, safe fish could also be used with tasty results. For the latest news on the safest types of fish to consume in your area, visit www.seafoodwatch.org.

CITRUS SLAW

2 tablespoons freshly squeezed lemon juice or lime juice

1 tablespoon honey

2 tablespoons diced red onion

1 tablespoon diced jalapeño

1 tablespoon extra-virgin olive oil

2 cups shredded cabbage

2 tablespoons chopped fresh cilantro

TACO FILLING

1 pound wild-caught cod, skinless and boneless

½ teaspoon sea salt

½ teaspoon ground cumin

½ teaspoon chili powder

1 teaspoon coconut oil

1 head butter lettuce or napa cabbage

Lime wedges, for garnish

1. Prepare the citrus slaw: In a large bowl, whisk together the lemon juice, honey, onion, jalapeño, and oil. Add the cabbage and cilantro and toss well to coat. For best flavor, allow the slaw to marinate for 1 to 2 hours before serving.

2. Prepare the taco filling: Cut the cod into 1-inch chunks and place them in a large bowl. Season with the salt, cumin, and chili powder and toss well to coat.

3. Melt the coconut oil in a large skillet over medium heat. Add the seasoned cod and sauté until the fish begins to flake and is thoroughly cooked, 8 to 10 minutes.

4. Use a slotted spoon to transfer the fish to lettuce leaves, then top with the citrus slaw. Serve immediately, garnished with lime wedges.

quinoa mushroom burgers

STARCH | (GF) (DF) (NF) (SF) (NS) (EF) (V) | *Serves 4*

These burgers may be vegetarian, but they're still a good source of protein thanks to the addition of quinoa. This gluten-free pseudograin is a complete source of protein, containing all nine essential amino acids. But unlike meat, it also packs a hefty dose of fiber with each serving (almost twice as much fiber as most grains!). While many veggie burgers use flour as a binder, this recipe calls for whole cooked quinoa, which won't spike your insulin levels the way flour can. Since these simple burgers are starch-based, you can enjoy them on your favorite bun or lettuce wrap, along with a side of Seasoned Sweet Potato Home Fries (page 92) for a satisfying, yet easily digested meal.

8 ounces mushrooms, sliced

2 carrots, chopped

3 celery stalks, chopped

½ cup quinoa

1 cup water

1 teaspoon coconut oil

½ yellow onion, chopped

2 cloves garlic, minced

1 teaspoon ground cumin

1 teaspoon chili powder

1 teaspoon sea salt

1. Preheat the oven to 350°F and line a large rimmed baking sheet with parchment paper.

2. Arrange the mushrooms, carrots, and celery in a single layer on the lined baking sheet and place in the oven to dry-roast for 30 minutes.

3. In the meantime, place the quinoa in a small saucepan and cover with the water. Bring to a boil, then cover, lower the heat, and cook for 15 minutes, until all of the water has been absorbed. Remove from the heat and set aside.

4. Melt the coconut oil in a skillet over medium heat and sauté the onion and garlic until tender, 8 to 10 minutes.

5. Transfer the cooked onion and garlic, roasted vegetables, and cooked quinoa to a large food processor fitted with an "S" blade. Add the cumin, chili powder, and salt and process until a uniform mixture is created. It should be sticky enough to easily form burger patties. When in doubt, err on the side of overprocessing this mixture, as it needs to be very sticky in order to not fall apart when baked.

6. Divide the mixture into 4 servings (about ½ cup each) and use your hands to shape patties that are ½ inch thick. Arrange them on the lined baking sheet and bake for 30 minutes. Remove from the oven and use a spatula to carefully flip them over (they will be delicate) and then return to the oven to bake for an additional 15 minutes. The burgers are done when the outside is crisp, but the inside is still tender. Serve warm.

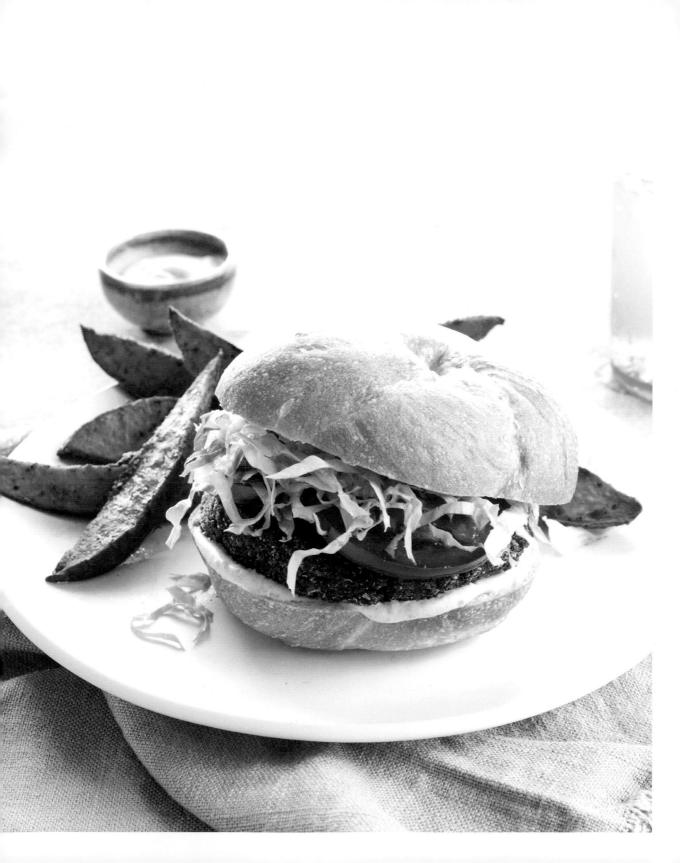

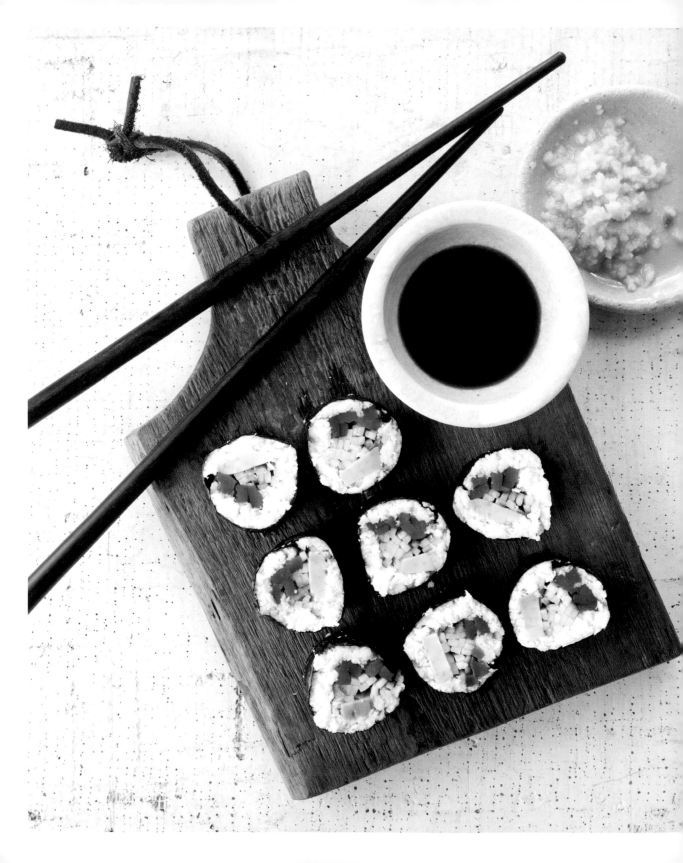

juice pulp sushi rolls

STARCH OR FRESH FRUIT | (GF) (DF) (NF) (NS) (EF) (V) | *Serves 4*

These rolls are a healthy way to get your sushi fix, while also repurposing the pulp left over from making fresh vegetable juice. In lieu of the sticky white rice found in regular sushi rolls, juice pulp provides a similar texture, without the starch content. Carrot pulp works particularly well as a rice substitute, as does jicama pulp. (Try juicing jicama—it makes a sweet drink that is reminiscent of horchata!) Paired with roasted red bell pepper, which acts as a slippery fishlike alternative, these rolls are sure to satisfy any sushi craving.

4 sheets nori (see note)

2 cups fresh juice pulp (see note, page 114)

2 Roasted Red Bell Peppers (page 181), sliced

1 avocado, pitted and sliced

½ cucumber, sliced into matchsticks

Sriracha sauce (optional)

Tamari, for dipping

Grated ginger, for dipping

1. Lay a nori sheet on top of a bamboo rolling mat or cutting board, with the textured side facing up. Working from the end closest to you, use your hands to spread out ½ cup of the juice pulp, pressing it evenly over the bottom half of the nori sheet.

2. Top the juice pulp with a horizontal row of roasted red pepper slices and avocado slices, followed by the cucumber matchsticks. Add a squirt of Sriracha sauce, if a spicy flavor is desired.

3. Starting from the bottom, roll the sheet up over the vegetables, being sure to tuck the vegetables in as you roll. (Using a bamboo rolling mat helps keep the roll tight.) Once you reach the end of the roll, dip your finger in water and run it along the end of the nori sheet to seal the roll. Enjoy the sushi roll as is, or slice it into smaller pieces, if desired. Repeat this process with the remaining 3 nori sheets to create 4 rolls in total.

4. Pour the tamari into a small bowl and top it with grated ginger for a quick and easy dipping sauce. Dip and enjoy!

NOTE: *Nori is an edible seaweed that is rich in plant protein and may help stabilize cholesterol levels. It's also a good source of iodine, with just one sushi roll containing over half of the recommended daily value for adults. Regular consumption of this particular seaweed has been associated with a lower risk of breast cancer in women.[2] Look for nori sheets in the Asian food section of your local grocery store.*

CONTINUED

When collecting juice pulp, be sure to juice your carrots or jicama first, so the pulp isn't affected by the other ingredients in the juice. (Lemon pulp would definitely affect the flavor of your sushi!) If you don't have a juicer, you can also create the "rice" by processing vegetables in a food processor or blender until a ricelike texture is achieved, and then squeezing the excess liquid out using a thin dish towel or nut milk bag.

make it soy-free Replace the tamari with coconut aminos.

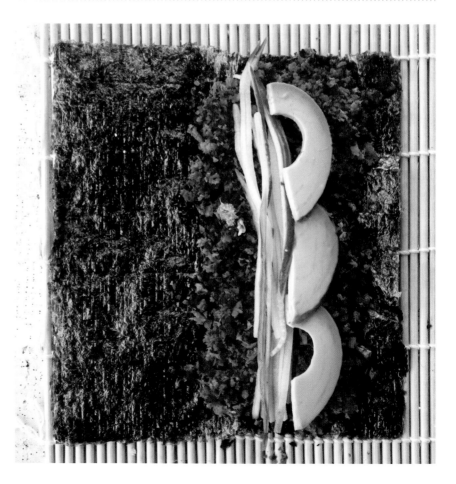

wild salmon sliders

ANIMAL PROTEIN | (GF) (DF) (NF) (NS) (EF) | *Serves 4*

These petite salmon burgers are a fun way to serve up this healthy fish, as they are handheld and appeal to all age groups. While most fish recipes require bread crumbs or eggs to create patties, this recipe relies on the simple use of a food processor to pulverize the fish, along with some tasty flavorings, into a mixture that will easily hold together when shaped with your hands. Compared to other fish, salmon has the highest content of omega-3 DHA fatty acids, which has been linked to promoting heart health and proper brain function. Serve them up in soft butter lettuce leaves with your favorite toppings for an easily digested and protein-packed meal.

1 pound wild-caught salmon, skin removed

1 red bell pepper, seeded and chopped

2 tablespoons chopped red onion

2 tablespoons finely chopped fresh parsley

2 cloves garlic, minced

1 tablespoon tamari

2 teaspoons Dijon mustard

½ teaspoon sea salt

Butter lettuce leaves or hamburger buns, for serving

1. Preheat the oven to 350°F and line a baking sheet with parchment paper.

2. In a large food processor fitted with an "S" blade, combine all of the ingredients except the lettuce leaves and process until the salmon is broken down, forming a mixture that easily sticks together.

3. Use a ¼-cup measuring cup to scoop the mixture and use your hands to shape a small patty about ½ inch thick. Repeat with the rest of the mixture, creating 8 to 10 patties, and then arrange them on the lined baking sheet. Bake until they are cooked through, 18 to 20 minutes. Serve warm in butter lettuce leaves, or on a bun if you prefer, with your favorite toppings.

NOTE: *If gluten-free recipes are not a priority for you, regular soy sauce can be substituted for tamari.*

make it soy-free Replace the tamari with coconut aminos.

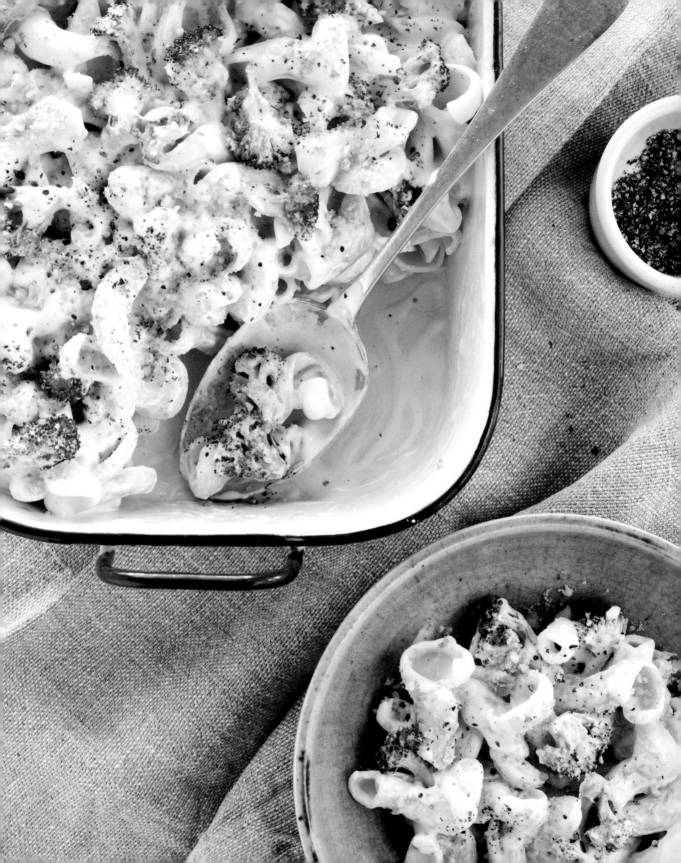

casseroles &
comfort food

When people hear the word *detox*, they may think that their favorite comfort foods are off the table for good. Not so, my friends! The following recipes have all of the comfort you crave, without the heavy ingredients and fillers that typically leave you feeling uncomfortable after eating. Whether you're in the mood for a slice of cheesy pizza, a box of Chinese takeout, or a plate of Thanksgiving stuffing with creamy mashed potatoes, this chapter has you covered. Get ready to dig in!

cheesy jalapeño casserole

ANIMAL PROTEIN | (GF) (NF) (SF) (NS) (EF) | *Serves 4 to 6*

This casserole is reminiscent of my mother's cheesy hash brown casserole, a dish that is always a hit with my family around the holidays. In lieu of frozen hash browns, this version relies on cooked spaghetti squash for a similar texture, while plain goat's milk yogurt provides a creamy base that is easier to digest than traditional sour cream. Diced jalapeños add an extra bite of flavor to this delicious casserole, but cooking them reduces their spiciness, for a generally appealing dish that the whole family can love.

1 teaspoon butter

½ yellow onion, chopped

2 jalapeños, seeded and finely diced

¼ cup chèvre (soft goat cheese)

1 cup plain goat's milk yogurt

1½ teaspoons sea salt

1 (3½-pound) Baked Spaghetti Squash (page 172)

1 ounce shredded raw goat's milk Cheddar

1. Preheat the oven to 350°F.

2. Melt the butter in a 10-inch skillet over medium heat. Add the onion and jalapeños and sauté until tender, 8 to 10 minutes.

3. In a large bowl, mix together the chèvre, yogurt, and salt. Add the sautéed onion and jalapeños and stir well. Using the tines of a fork, scrape the cooked spaghetti squash flesh (about 5 cups) into the bowl and stir well to mix.

4. Transfer the mixture to a 3½-quart casserole dish and top with the Cheddar. Bake until the edges are golden, 35 to 40 minutes. Serve warm.

make it omnivore-friendly Add high-quality meat to this dish.

mexican butternut pilaf

STARCH | (GF) (DF) (NF) (SF) (NS) (EF) (V) | *Serves 4 to 6*

This warm dish is reminiscent of Mexican rice, but with far more texture and flavor. When briefly pulsed in a food processor, raw butternut squash becomes an amazingly quick and easy rice substitute, offering a slightly sweet flavor that is perfectly balanced by the spicy additions to this dish. Since this recipe is entirely vegetable-based, it makes quite a large quantity to accommodate 4 to 6 people. Be sure to use a large stockpot or enameled Dutch oven to squeeze all of those delicious vegetables in!

1 (2½-pound) butternut squash, peeled and cubed

1 teaspoon coconut oil

1 yellow onion, chopped

1 red bell pepper, chopped

1 jalapeño, diced (seeds optional)

1 pound tomatoes, chopped

2 cloves garlic

2 teaspoons ground cumin

1½ teaspoons chili powder

1½ teaspoons sea salt

Sliced avocado, for garnish

Chopped fresh cilantro, for garnish

1. In a large food processor fitted with an "S" blade, briefly process the cubed butternut squash until a ricelike texture is achieved. Set aside.

2. Melt the coconut oil in a large stockpot or enameled Dutch oven over medium heat. Add the onion, bell pepper, and jalapeño and sauté until the onion is translucent, about 8 minutes.

3. Add the tomatoes, garlic, and butternut squash "rice," along with the ground cumin, chili powder, and salt. Stir well to combine, and then lower the heat, cover, and cook until the butternut "rice" is tender, about 10 minutes. Stir again, add any extra seasoning to taste, and serve warm with sliced avocado and fresh cilantro on top.

make it more filling Add 1½ cups cooked beans or lentils for a more filling yet still properly combined meal.

cauliflower fried "rice"

ANIMAL PROTEIN | (GF) (DF) (NF) (NS) | *Serves 4 to 6*

This is my favorite dish to introduce to people who are new to healthier eating, as it tastes incredibly similar to real Chinese takeout, while being almost entirely vegetable-based. When briefly pulsed in a food processor, raw cauliflower becomes surprisingly ricelike and is almost undetectable when sautéed with aromatic garlic, ginger, and tamari. The fluffy bites of egg are my favorite part of any fried rice dish, but the eggs can be easily omitted to make this recipe vegan-friendly.

1 (2½-pound) head cauliflower, chopped into florets

2 tablespoons coconut oil

½ yellow onion, chopped

3 celery stalks, chopped

2 carrots, chopped

2 cups chopped broccoli florets

2 cloves garlic, minced

1 teaspoon minced ginger

6 eggs, beaten

⅓ cup tamari

Sea salt

1. In a large food processor fitted with an "S" blade, briefly pulse the cauliflower florets into a ricelike consistency. Be careful not to overprocess, as you don't want the "rice" to be too fine. (Alternatively, you could grate the cauliflower on a box grater.) Set aside.

2. Melt 1 tablespoon of the coconut oil in a large saucepan or enameled Dutch oven over medium heat. Add the onion, celery, and carrots and sauté until slightly tender, about 5 minutes. Add the broccoli, garlic, and ginger and cover. Cook for another 5 minutes, until the broccoli is bright green.

3. Melt the remaining 1 tablespoon of coconut oil in a separate skillet over medium heat. Add the eggs and scramble until they are softly cooked and fluffy.

4. Add the scrambled eggs, cauliflower "rice," and tamari to the saucepan full of cooked vegetables and stir well, cooking until the cauliflower "rice" is hot and tender. Season with sea salt to taste and then serve immediately.

make it vegan Omit the eggs.

make it soy-free Replace the tamari with coconut aminos.

make it omnivore-friendly Add high-quality meat to this dish for a properly combined meal.

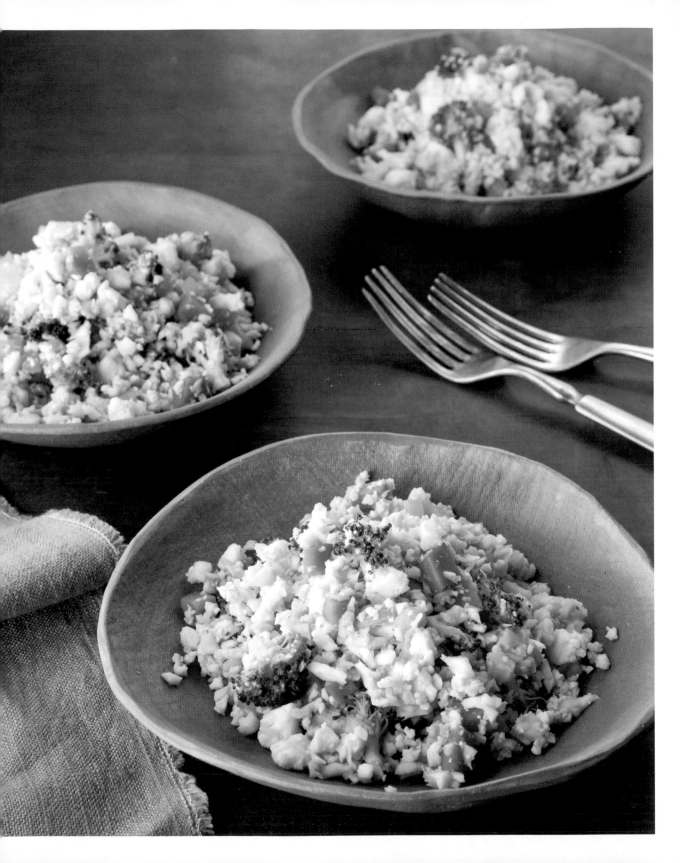

creamy pumpkin & sage pasta

STARCH | (GF) (DF) (SF) (NS) (EF) (V) | *Serves 4 to 6*

This dairy-free pasta dish is a tasty addition to an autumn menu. Cooked pumpkin and fresh sage quickly combine to make a savory sauce that will digest easily with your favorite high-quality pasta, without the need for heavy cream or butter. Serve with a sprinkling of nutritional yeast, if desired, to add an extra "cheesy" flavor to this comforting meal.

1 teaspoon coconut oil

1 yellow onion, chopped

3 cloves garlic, minced

1¾ cups cooked pumpkin puree or 1 (15-ounce) can pumpkin puree

1 cup Homemade Almond Milk (page 178)

1 tablespoon minced fresh sage leaves

1½ teaspoons sea salt

1 pound gluten-free pasta

Nutritional yeast, for garnish (optional)

1. Melt the coconut oil in a skillet over medium heat. Add the onion and sauté until tender, 8 to 10 minutes. Add the garlic and sauté until fragrant, about 1 minute.

2. Transfer the onion and garlic to a high-speed blender and add the pumpkin puree, almond milk, sage, and salt. Blend until completely smooth and set aside.

3. Prepare the pasta according to the package directions, then drain and return the pasta to the stockpot over medium heat. Add in the pumpkin sauce and stir well, until the pasta and sauce are hot. Serve immediately, with a sprinkling of nutritional yeast on top.

NOTE: *For a grain-free pasta dish, serve this sauce over Baked Spaghetti Squash (page 172), but be sure to season with additional salt to balance out the naturally sweet flavor of the squash "noodles."*

oil-free walnut pesto pasta

NUT/SEED/DRIED FRUIT | GF DF SF NS EF V | *Serves 4 to 6*

This pesto is one of the easiest meals in my repertoire, as the sauce can be whipped up in less than 5 minutes, with just a cutting board and a blender. Traditional pesto recipes require plenty of olive oil, cheese, and toasted pine nuts, but this recipe gets its buttery texture and flavor from a combination of raw walnuts and fresh zucchini, without the need for any added oils. The result is a creamy pesto that's lower in fat, higher in fiber, and still bursting with flavor. Serve over raw or sautéed zucchini "noodles" for an easily digested meal or enjoy as a dip with your favorite raw crudités.

PESTO

1 cup diced zucchini

1 cup fresh basil leaves, tightly packed

3 cloves garlic, minced

½ cup raw walnut halves

¼ cup water

2 tablespoons freshly squeezed lemon juice

½ teaspoon sea salt

4 to 6 large zucchini, peeled

1 teaspoon coconut oil (optional)

1 cup cherry tomatoes, halved

Raw pine nuts, for garnish (optional)

1. Prepare the pesto: Combine all of the pesto ingredients in a high-speed blender and blend until completely smooth. For a chunkier texture, instead use the pulse function on your blender or food processor to gently mix the ingredients together.

2. Use a spiralizer or vegetable peeler to create "noodles" out of the peeled zucchini. For a warm dish, melt the coconut oil in a large skillet over medium heat and sauté the zucchini "noodles" and tomatoes until tender, 8 to 10 minutes. Add in the pesto and stir quickly, just enough to warm the sauce, about 1 minute. Serve warm, with a sprinkle of pine nuts. For a cold dish, simply toss the raw zucchini "noodles" with the prepared pesto and top with the tomatoes and pine nuts.

NOTE: *You can easily freeze sauces like this one for a convenient future meal. Simply pour the sauce into ice cube trays to freeze, creating cubes that can be easily thawed and portioned for one or more people. Thaw the sauce cubes directly in a skillet with your pasta or veggies of choice, and your whole meal will be ready in less than 10 minutes.*

southwest stuffed sweet potatoes

STARCH | GF DF NF SF NS EF V | *Serves 4*

Instead of the traditional butter and brown sugar toppings, these baked sweet potatoes are dressed with a savory mix of sautéed onions, peppers, tomatoes, and spinach, with a kick of spice for some Southwestern flair. Sweet potatoes, which are also commonly labeled as yams, contain almost twice as much fiber as other potatoes and are bursting with vitamin B_6, which may promote heart health. These stuffed spuds can be easily reheated in the oven, so feel free to make a double batch and freeze the extras for a convenient meal during the week.

4 sweet potatoes

2 teaspoons coconut oil

1 red onion, chopped

1 red bell pepper, seeded and chopped

1 jalapeño, diced (seeds optional)

2 cloves garlic, minced

2 tomatoes, chopped

½ teaspoon cumin

½ teaspoon chili powder

½ teaspoon sea salt

2 cups fresh spinach

1 avocado, pitted

Chopped fresh cilantro, for garnish

1. Preheat the oven to 350°F.

2. Pierce the skin of the sweet potatoes several times with a fork to vent, then rub the skins with 1 teaspoon of the coconut oil. Place the potatoes on a baking sheet and bake until tender, 45 to 60 minutes.

3. Melt the remaining 1 teaspoon of coconut oil in a skillet over medium heat. Add the onion, bell pepper, and jalapeño and sauté for 5 minutes. Add the garlic and tomatoes along with the cumin, chili powder, and salt and sauté for another 5 minutes, allowing the liquid from the tomatoes to evaporate. Finally, add in the fresh spinach, sautéing just long enough for the leaves to wilt.

4. Remove the baked sweet potatoes from the oven, cut in half lengthwise, and lightly sprinkle with sea salt. Spoon the sautéed vegetable filling over the potatoes, then top each with diced ripe avocado and a sprinkling of cilantro. Serve warm.

make it more filling Add 1½ cups cooked beans or lentils for a more filling yet still properly combined meal.

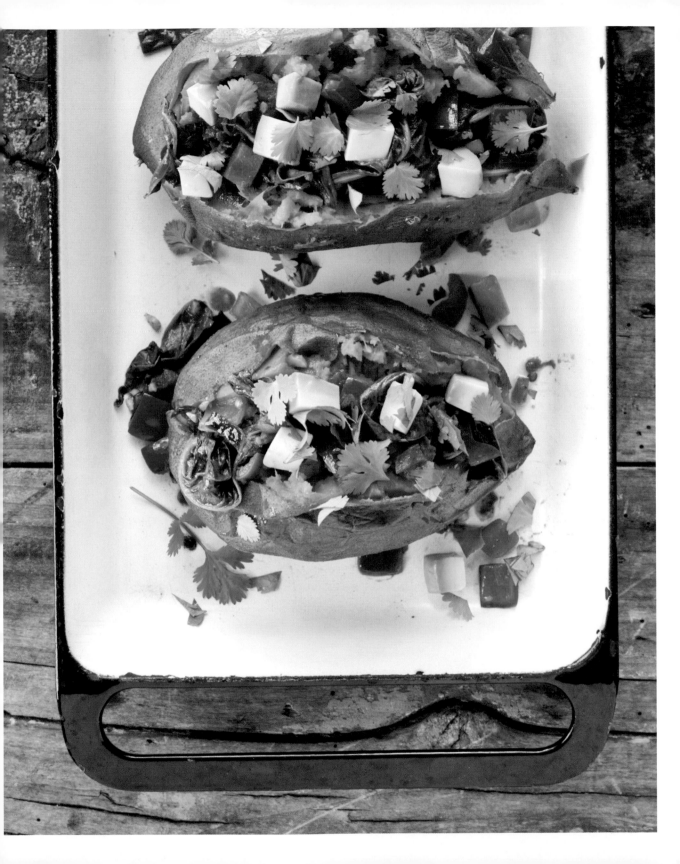

baked stuffing loaf

ANIMAL PROTEIN | (GF) (DF) (NF) (SF) (NS) | *Serves 4*

This dish is a little labor-intensive, but it features all of the flavors of Thanksgiving stuffing that you love, without the butter or bread that traditionally makes it so heavy. Dry-roasted vegetables are key to this uniquely healthy stuffing, as they help create an appealing texture without adding too much moisture to the mix. Combined with protein-rich eggs, this dish is a cross between stuffing and meatloaf and is a comforting holiday dish you can enjoy any time of year.

1 pound cauliflower florets, chopped (about ½ head)

3 large carrots, chopped

3 celery stalks, chopped

8 ounces mushrooms, sliced

1 teaspoon coconut oil

½ yellow onion, chopped

4 cloves garlic, minced

3 eggs

2 teaspoons fresh thyme leaves

1 tablespoon minced fresh sage leaves

1½ teaspoons sea salt

Mushroom Gravy (page 178), for serving

1. Preheat the oven to 350°F. Line two rimmed baking sheets and a standard loaf pan with parchment paper. Arrange the cauliflower, carrots, celery, and mushrooms in a single layer on each baking sheet and dry-roast for 30 minutes.

2. In the meantime, melt the coconut oil in a skillet over medium heat. Add the onion and garlic and sauté until tender, 8 to 10 minutes.

3. Remove the dry-roasted vegetables from the oven and transfer them to a large food processor fitted with an "S" blade. Add the cooked onions and garlic, eggs, thyme, sage, and salt and pulse several times to combine, leaving as much texture as you desire.

4. Pour the mixture into the loaf pan and use a spatula to smooth the top. Bake until the center looks cooked through, about 1 hour. Slice and serve warm, with Mushroom Gravy over the top.

make it vegan Omit the eggs and simply stir together the pulsed vegetables, cooked vegetables, and seasonings for a loose stuffing that will digest easily with any meal.

make it omnivore-friendly Serve this stuffing with roasted turkey for a properly combined holiday meal.

enchilada stuffed cabbage rolls

STARCH | (GF) (DF) (NF) (SF) (NS) (EF) (V) | *Serves 4 to 6*

These stuffed cabbage rolls are the perfect way to satisfy a craving for enchiladas, without the use of greasy corn tortillas or excess cheese. Sweet potatoes and black beans make a delicious and filling combination, particularly when seasoned with Mexican spices and smothered in a rich enchilada sauce. Beans tend to be difficult to digest, due to their natural starch and protein content, but wrapping them in tender savoy cabbage leaves makes this meal lighter on digestion and offers plenty of soluble fiber and minerals, like magnesium and folate. Top off these rolls with a scoop of Classic Guacamole (page 94) for a satisfying and nourishing meal.

1 pound sweet potatoes, cut into 1-inch chunks

1 teaspoon coconut oil

1 yellow onion, chopped

2 cloves garlic, minced

1½ cups cooked black beans or 1 (15-ounce) can black beans, rinsed and drained

1 teaspoon ground cumin

1 teaspoon sea salt

3 cups Fresh Enchilada Sauce (page 176) or store-bought enchilada sauce

6 to 8 savoy cabbage leaves

1. Preheat the oven to 350°F.

2. Place the sweet potato chunks in a steamer basket fitted in a small saucepan filled with a couple of inches of water. Bring the water to a boil, then cover and lower the heat, steaming the potatoes until tender, about 10 minutes. Drain and set aside.

3. Melt the coconut oil in a skillet over medium heat. Add the onion and sauté until tender, 8 to 10 minutes. Add the garlic and sauté until fragrant, about 1 minute. Stir in the black beans, cumin, and salt and sauté until heated through.

4. Add the steamed sweet potatoes to the skillet and use the back of a fork to mash them into the cooked black bean mixture, leaving as much texture as you like.

5. Pour 1 cup of the enchilada sauce into the bottom of a 9 by 13-inch pan. Fill each of the cabbage leaves with the sweet potato filling and then wrap the leaves around the filling, creating a roll. Arrange the filled cabbage rolls in a single layer in the pan. Pour the remaining 2 cups of enchilada sauce over the top and bake for 35 to 40 minutes, until the cabbage rolls are tender and the sauce is piping hot. Serve warm.

NOTE: *These cabbage roll-ups are a versatile way to enjoy the flavor of enchiladas, without creating a digestive burden. If you want a more traditional enchilada, skip the sweet potato mixture and use your favorite meat and cheese filling instead.*

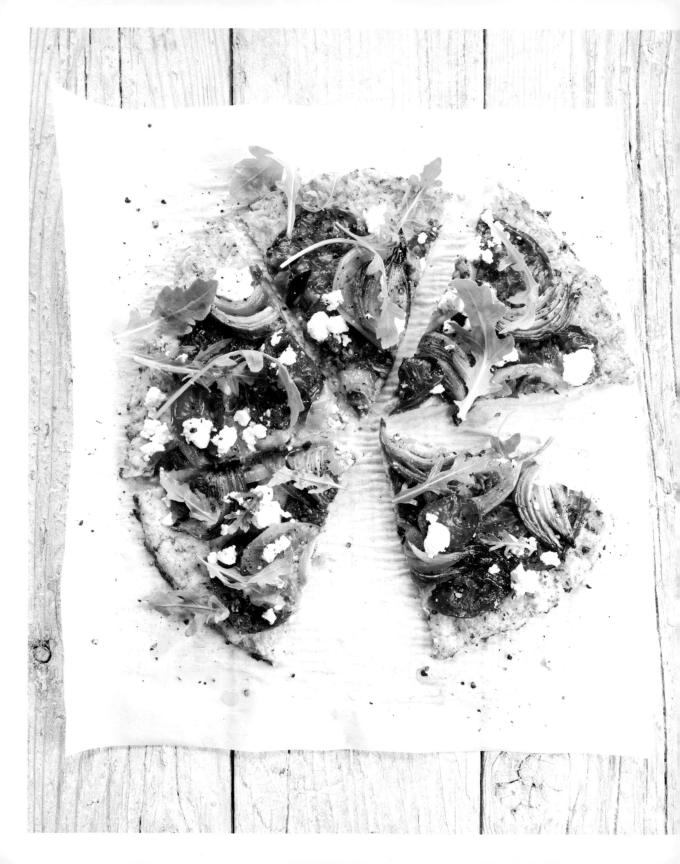

cauliflower flatbread pizza

ANIMAL PROTEIN | (GF) (NF) (SF) (NS) | *Serves 2 to 4*

Traditional pizza can be a digestive disaster, since it usually combines a starchy crust with gluey cheese, but this cauliflower version digests seamlessly and is just as satisfying. The key to getting a truly flatbreadlike crust is wringing out the cauliflower thoroughly, removing as much moisture as possible. You'll be amazed at the dry texture of this low-carb and protein-rich alternative, which can be enjoyed with your favorite pizza toppings or used as a flatbread for sandwiches. Because this process can be a bit labor-intensive, you may want to double or triple this recipe and freeze the extras for a quick pizza night in the future.

2 pounds frozen cauliflower florets, thawed

1 egg, lightly beaten

½ cup chèvre (soft goat cheese)

2 teaspoons dried oregano

1 teaspoon dried basil

½ teaspoon sea salt

1. Preheat the oven to 400°F and line a baking sheet with parchment paper.

2. In a large food processor fitted with an "S" blade, pulse the cauliflower florets several times, until a ricelike consistency is achieved. Pour the cauliflower into the center of a thin dish towel, then twist it up and use your hands to firmly wring out moisture. Quite a lot of liquid should be released, leaving you with a dry lump of cauliflower pulp.

3. Place the cauliflower pulp in a large mixing bowl and mix in the egg, chèvre, oregano, basil, and salt, stirring well to create a uniform mixture.

4. Transfer the cauliflower mixture to the baking sheet and use your hands to press the crust firmly into a large circular or rectangular crust, about ¼ inch thick. Be sure to pack the cauliflower mixture together firmly and evenly, leaving no thin spots where the crust may crack.

5. Bake for 30 minutes, until the top is dry and golden, then carefully flip the crust over and bake for another 10 minutes. Use immediately as a pizza crust or allow the flatbread to cool and slice it to use as sandwich bread.

6. To complete the pizza, add your favorite sauce and toppings and then bake for another 10 minutes at 400°F, until the topping are heated thoroughly. Slice and serve hot.

make it omnivore-friendly Add your favorite high-quality meat toppings.

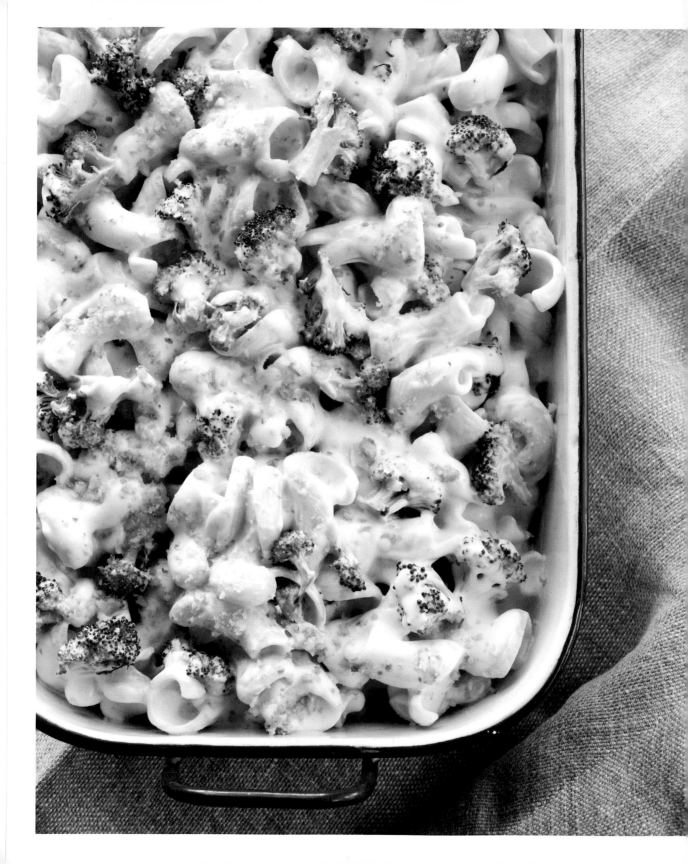

vegan mac 'n' cheese with roasted broccoli

NUT/SEED/DRIED FRUIT | (GF) (DF) (SF) (NS) (EF) (V) | *Serves 4 to 6*

Those of us who can't, or choose not to, consume dairy need not miss out on this childhood favorite. Made from creamy cashews, this vegan cheese sauce gets its cheesy flavor from a combination of lemon juice, salt, and nutritional yeast, which is a complete source of protein and loaded with B vitamins. Soaking the cashews in water before blending makes them easier to blend, and also easier to digest, but don't soak them for longer than 2 hours, as they may develop a slimy texture if left too long. Take this dish to the next level by stirring in oven-roasted broccoli, which adds an appealing texture and flavor, not to mention an extra dose of nutrition. Serve with Walnut "Parmesan" for a surprisingly authentic and delicious bread crumb–like topping.

1 (3½-pound) Baked Spaghetti Squash (page 172)

ROASTED BROCCOLI
½ pound broccoli florets, roughly chopped (about 4 cups)

1 tablespoon melted coconut oil

¼ teaspoon sea salt

CHEESE SAUCE
1½ cups whole raw cashews, soaked for up to 2 hours, drained, and rinsed well (see page 28)

¾ cup Homemade Almond Milk (page 178)

¼ cup nutritional yeast

2 tablespoons freshly squeezed lemon juice

2 teaspoons sea salt

½ teaspoon garlic powder

½ teaspoon Dijon mustard

Walnut "Parmesan" (page 181), for garnish

1. Preheat the oven to 400°F. Prepare the spaghetti squash according to the recipe on page 172 and bake for 40 minutes. While the squash is baking, prepare the roasted broccoli.

2. Prepare the broccoli: In a large bowl, combine the broccoli, coconut oil, and salt and toss well to coat. Arrange the broccoli in a single layer on a rimmed baking sheet. After the squash has baked for 40 minutes, lower the heat to 350°F, and add the broccoli to the oven. Bake the squash and broccoli for 20 minutes more, until the outer skin of the squash has developed a light brown coloring and can be easily pierced with a fork and the broccoli is tender and starting to brown.

3. Prepare the cheese sauce: Combine the cashews, almond milk, nutritional yeast, lemon juice, salt, garlic powder, and mustard in a high-speed blender and blend until completely smooth and creamy.

4. Remove the spaghetti squash from the oven and carefully scrape the cooked flesh into a serving dish, creating spaghetti noodle–like strands. Immediately pour the cheese sauce over the piping-hot "pasta," stir in the roasted broccoli, and serve right away with a sprinkle of Walnut "Parmesan."

VARIATION: Use 1 pound of high-quality dried pasta in place of the spaghetti squash. Prepare the roasted broccoli and cheese sauce as described above, then prepare the pasta according to the instructions on the package, reserving ½ cup of the cooking water to stir in with the cheese sauce. The sauce isn't properly combined when served with traditional grain-based pasta, but it makes an excellent transitional meal for those missing mainstream comfort food.

italian "meatloaf" muffins

ANIMAL PROTEIN | GF NF SF NS | *Makes 12 muffins*

These vegetarian muffins are incredibly meatlike, without the need for any processed soy substitutes. Mushrooms tend to provide a meaty quality to any dish, and when paired with vegetables that have been pulsed in a food processor, the texture becomes similar to that of ground beef. Enjoy them as "meatballs" over Baked Spaghetti Squash (page 172) or on their own with a topping of marinara sauce for a satisfying Italian-inspired meal.

3 carrots, chopped

3 celery stalks, chopped

1 yellow onion, chopped

1 teaspoon butter

4 cloves garlic, minced

1 pound mushrooms, sliced

2 teaspoons dried oregano

2 teaspoons dried basil

¾ teaspoon salt

½ cup grated sheep's milk pecorino

2 eggs, beaten

Easy Marinara Sauce (page 174) or store-bought marinara, for serving

1. Preheat the oven to 350°F. Line a large baking sheet with parchment paper and line a standard muffin tin with silicone or parchment baking cups.

2. Arrange the carrots, celery, and onion in a single layer on the baking sheet and dry-roast for 30 minutes.

3. Meanwhile, melt the butter in a large skillet over medium heat. Add the garlic and mushrooms and sauté until tender, 6 to 8 minutes.

4. Using a slotted spoon, transfer the sautéed mushrooms and garlic to a large food processor fitted with an "S" blade. Add the roasted vegetables, oregano, basil, and salt and pulse 3 to 5 times to combine.

5. Add the grated cheese and beaten eggs and pulse another 3 to 5 times, just enough to combine but still leaving some texture to the mix.

6. Divide the batter among the 12 lined muffin cups and bake until the edges are lightly golden and the center is firm, 35 to 40 minutes. Serve immediately, with warm marinara sauce over the top of each muffin.

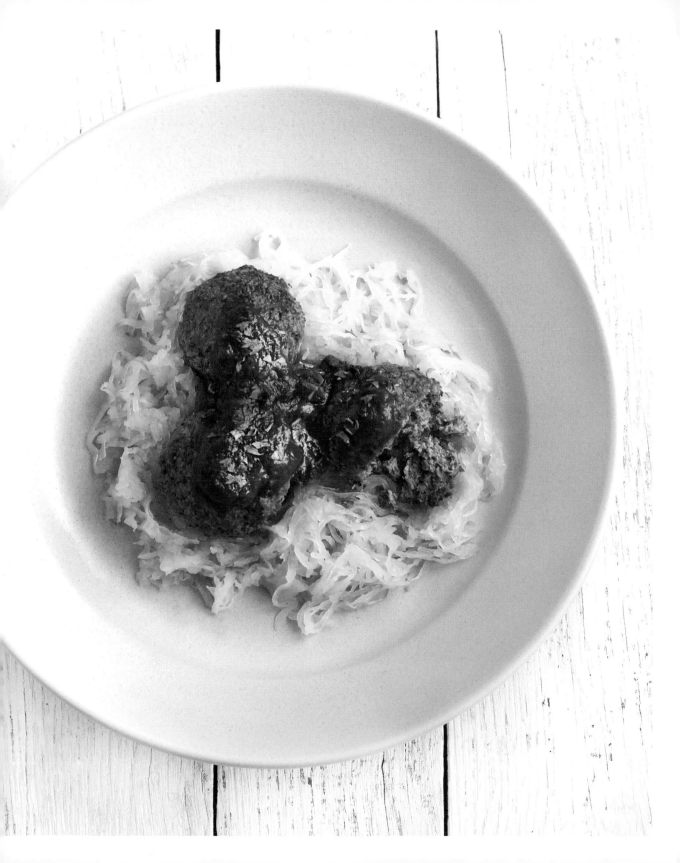

easy coconut curry

STARCH | (GF) (DF) (NF) (EF) (V) | *Serves 4*

This curry dish is one of my family's favorite weeknight meals, as it comes together in just about 20 minutes and works well with any vegetables you have on hand. On especially busy nights, I like to use a bag of frozen assorted vegetables, which will thaw and cook directly in this sauce with virtually no prep work required.

CURRY SAUCE

1 teaspoon coconut oil

½ yellow onion, chopped

2 cloves garlic, minced

1 teaspoon fresh minced
   ginger

1½ tablespoons curry
   powder

1¾ cups coconut milk

1 tablespoon tamari

1 tablespoon maple syrup

1 pound assorted
   vegetables, chopped
   (fresh or frozen)

2 sweet potatoes, chopped

Sea salt and pepper

Cooked quinoa or Basic
   Cauliflower "Rice"
   (page 172), for serving

1. Prepare the curry sauce: Melt the coconut oil in a large stockpot or Dutch oven over medium heat. Add the onion and sauté until tender, about 8 minutes. Add the garlic and ginger and sauté until fragrant, about 1 minute. Add the curry powder, coconut milk, tamari, and syrup and whisk well to combine.

2. Add the vegetables and sweet potatoes to the sauce and bring the mixture to a boil. Cover and lower the heat, allowing the vegetables to cook until fork-tender, about 15 minutes. Season with salt and pepper and serve warm over a bed of cooked quinoa.

NOTE: *Depending on your time and budget, you can use Fresh Coconut Milk (page 175) or the canned version for this recipe, both with great results. When opting for the convenience of canned coconut milk, be sure to look for cans that are labeled BPA-free.*

make it soy-free Replace the tamari with coconut aminos.

make it sugar-free Replace the maple syrup with stevia, to taste.

pantry pad thai

NUT/SEED/DRIED FRUIT | (GF) (DF) (EF) | *Serves 4*

This simplified version of the popular Thai dish covers all of the flavors you've come to love, using ingredients you most likely already have in your pantry. Though tamarind paste is called for in many traditional recipes, it's not an ingredient that most of us use on a regular basis, so this dish gets its sour flavor from fresh lime juice instead. If you're not familiar with Sriracha, it is a spicy sauce made from red chile peppers and garlic that is often served with Thai and Vietnamese cuisine. I like to keep it in our refrigerator door as an easy way to add spice to any dish.

PAD THAI SAUCE

¼ cup Raw Almond Butter (page 179)

¼ cup tamari

3 tablespoons freshly squeezed lime juice

3 tablespoons clover honey

1 to 2 teaspoons Sriracha sauce

1 teaspoon coconut oil

4 cups shredded cabbage

4 cloves garlic, minced

2 carrots, julienned or shredded

4 green onions, sliced (green and white parts separated)

1 (3½-pound) Baked Spaghetti Squash (page 172)

½ cup slivered raw almonds

1 cup mung bean sprouts (optional)

1. Prepare the sauce: In a medium bowl, combine the almond butter, tamari, lime juice, honey, and Sriracha and whisk well. Set aside.

2. Melt the coconut oil in a large stockpot or Dutch oven over medium heat. Add the cabbage, garlic, carrots, and the white parts of the onions and sauté until tender, about 5 minutes. Add in the baked spaghetti squash "noodles" and stir well to heat thoroughly.

3. Turn off the heat and quickly stir in the sauce, coating the vegetables well. Adjust the flavor by adding more tamari or Sriracha to taste, then toss in the green parts of the onions, the almonds, and the mung bean sprouts. Stir well and serve immediately.

make it vegan Replace the honey with maple syrup.

make it sugar-free Replace the honey with stevia, to taste.

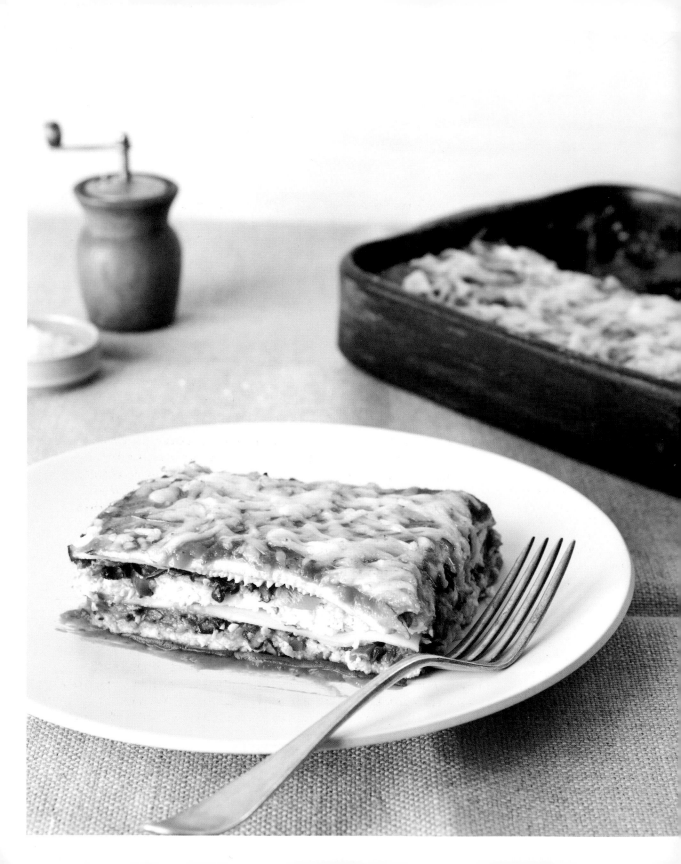

zucchini lasagna

ANIMAL PROTEIN | GF NF SF NS | *Serves 4*

Healthy or not, lasagna tends to be a labor-intensive dish. This zucchini version is no more difficult to prepare than the traditional kind and it tastes just as delicious, without weighing you down. The key to avoiding a watery result is salting the zucchini "noodles," to draw out any excess moisture, and then rinsing and patting them dry. Featuring unique vegetable fillings, like cauliflower "ricotta" and mushroom "meat," this dish is loaded with nutrition and is sure to satisfy your lasagna cravings. It may even surprise the skeptics in your life!

4 zucchini
   (about ½ pound)
Sea salt
1½ cups Easy Marinara
   Sauce (page 174)
Shredded goat's milk
   Cheddar, for topping
   (optional)

CAULIFLOWER "RICOTTA"
1 pound frozen cauliflower,
   thawed
2 eggs, lightly beaten
½ cup chèvre
   (soft goat cheese)
1 teaspoon dried oregano
½ teaspoon sea salt

MUSHROOM "MEAT"
1 teaspoon butter
½ yellow onion, chopped
2 cloves garlic, minced
8 ounces mushrooms,
   roughly chopped
½ teaspoon sea salt

1. Preheat the oven to 350°F.

2. Thinly slice the zucchini lengthwise, about ⅛ inch thick, using a sharp knife or mandoline slicer. (There's no need to peel the zucchini, unless you want to.) Use your hands to gently rub the "noodles" with a generous pinch of sea salt and then set aside in a large bowl to sweat while you prepare the fillings.

3. Prepare the cauliflower "ricotta": Process the thawed cauliflower in a food processor fitted with an "S" blade, to create a ricelike texture. Transfer the cauliflower to a thin dish towel, then twist it up and use your hands to firmly squeeze out the moisture. A lot of liquid should be released, leaving a very dry cauliflower pulp. Place the pulp in a large bowl and mix in the eggs, chèvre, oregano, and salt. Set aside.

4. Prepare the mushroom "meat": In a skillet over medium heat, melt the butter. Add the onion and sauté for 5 minutes. Add the garlic, mushrooms, and salt and sauté until the mushrooms are tender, 6 to 8 minutes.

5. Rinse and drain the zucchini "noodles," then pat them dry with a towel.

6. To assemble the lasagna, spread a thin layer of marinara sauce across the bottom of a 9-inch square dish to prevent sticking, then arrange several zucchini "noodles" to cover the sauce, overlapping slightly. Spoon half of the cauliflower mixture over the top of the zucchini layer, distributing it evenly. Use a slotted spoon to sprinkle half of the mushroom mixture over the cauliflower layer, and then spoon a bit more marinara sauce over the top. Add another layer

CONTINUED

of zucchini, then repeat the process with the remaining cauliflower and mushroom layers. Add a final layer of zucchini and top them off with a layer of marinara sauce.

7. Bake for 60 minutes. Sprinkle a layer of shredded cheese over the top of the lasagna during the final 10 minutes of baking, giving it just enough time to melt. Remove from the oven and allow the dish to sit for 20 minutes before cutting and serving.

make it omnivore-friendly Though this dish is already rather meatlike, you can add cooked ground beef to the mushroom mixture, if you desire. Be sure to drain the cooked meat well to avoid a soggy result.

creamy cauliflower alfredo

NEUTRAL | GF DF SF NS EF V | *Serves 4*

This Alfredo sauce is as guilt-free as it gets. In lieu of the heavy cream, butter, and cheese found in the original version, this creamy sauce gets its smooth and velvety texture from pureed cauliflower, which means it can be served over any type of pasta you like, without hindering digestion. When poured over homemade zucchini "noodles," you can still add a generous sprinkling of grated Pecorino Romano for an authentic cheesy flavor, without consuming a heavy amount of dairy. For a dairy-free topping, try using a spoonful of Walnut "Parmesan" (page 181), instead.

2 teaspoons coconut oil

3 cloves garlic, minced

1 pound cauliflower florets (about ½ head)

1 cup water

½ cup Homemade Almond Milk (page 178)

1 teaspoon sea salt

4 large zucchini, peeled

Freshly ground black pepper

1. Melt 1 teaspoon of the coconut oil in a saucepan over medium heat. Add the garlic and sauté just until fragrant, about 1 minute. Add the cauliflower and water (the water doesn't have to cover the cauliflower) and bring the water to a boil. Lower the heat and cover, simmering until the cauliflower is very soft and tender, about 15 minutes.

2. Transfer the cooked cauliflower mixture to a high-speed blender, add the almond milk and salt, and then blend until very smooth. (When blending hot liquids, be sure to remove the plastic cap from the blender lid and cover the opening with a dish towel to allow steam to escape and prevent burns.)

3. Use a spiralizer or vegetable peeler to create zucchini "noodles." Melt the remaining 1 teaspoon of coconut oil in a large stockpot or Dutch oven. Add the zucchini and sauté until tender, 8 to 10 minutes. Pour the cauliflower sauce into the pan and toss well. Once the sauce is piping hot, serve immediately, with freshly ground black pepper and any other desired toppings.

make it omnivore-friendly When served over zucchini "noodles," this meal would still be easily digested with a serving of high-quality meat.

maple mustard glazed salmon

ANIMAL PROTEIN | (GF) (DF) (NF) (SF) (EF) | *Serves 4*

This is by far one of the easiest ways to prepare salmon, and one of the tastiest, too. This meaty fish provides a significant serving of omega-3 fatty acids, which are thought to play an important role in reducing inflammation throughout the body, and they may also promote brain health. Calling for a simple two-ingredient glaze, this healthy meal comes together in minutes.

1 pound wild-caught salmon fillets (about 4 ounces per person)

Sea salt

2 tablespoons maple syrup

2 tablespoons Dijon mustard

1. Preheat the broiler and place the oven rack about 6 inches below the heat source.

2. Arrange the salmon on a baking sheet, skin side down, and sprinkle the top generously with salt. In a small bowl, mix together the maple syrup and Dijon, then pour the mixture over the salmon fillets.

3. Broil until the salmon flakes easily with a fork, 10 to 12 minutes. Serve warm.

NOTE: *Select wild-caught salmon to avoid the antibiotics and higher levels of toxins often found in the farm-raised variety. Look for Alaskan salmon whenever possible, as it is always wild-caught.*

make it sugar-free Replace the maple syrup with stevia, to taste.

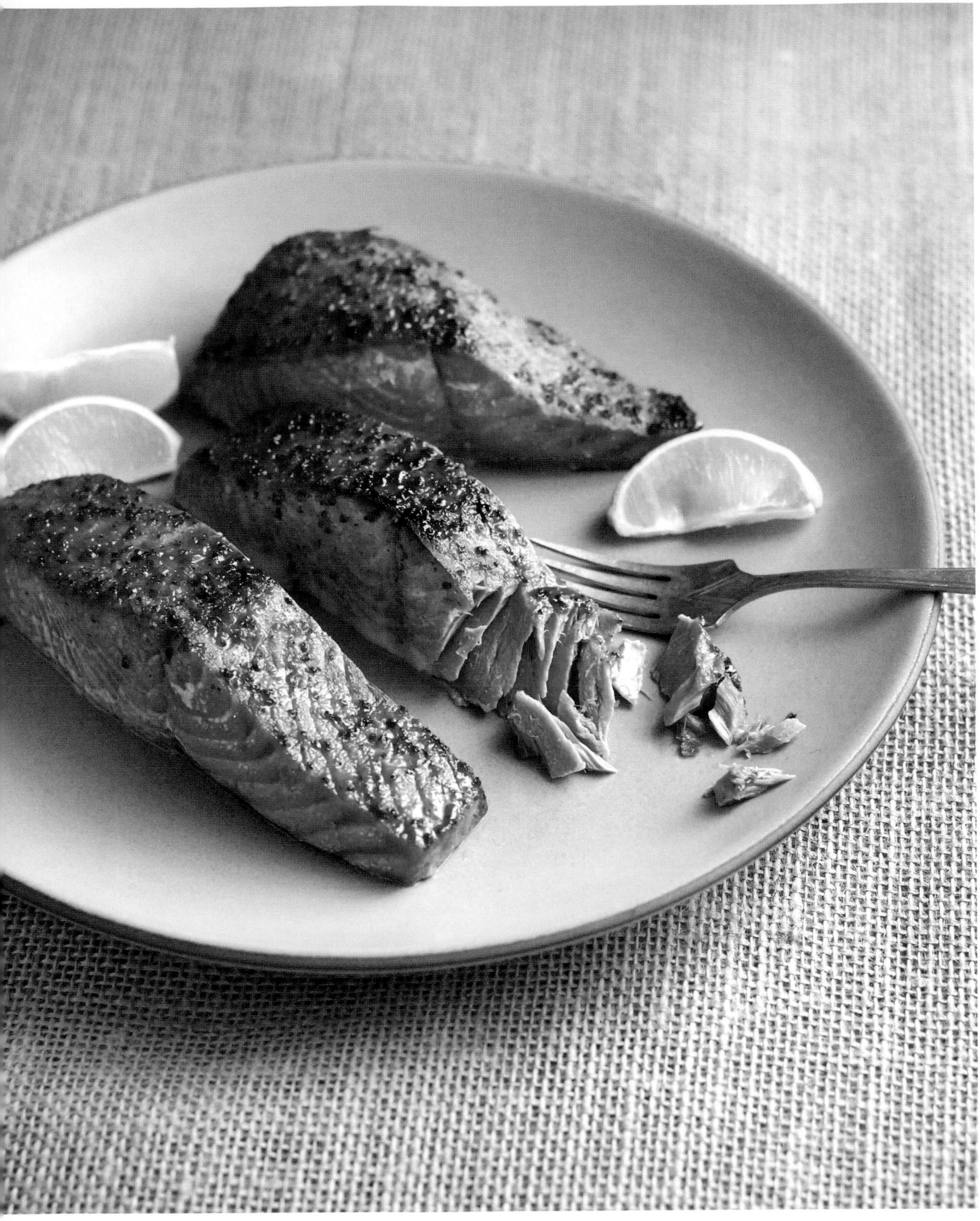

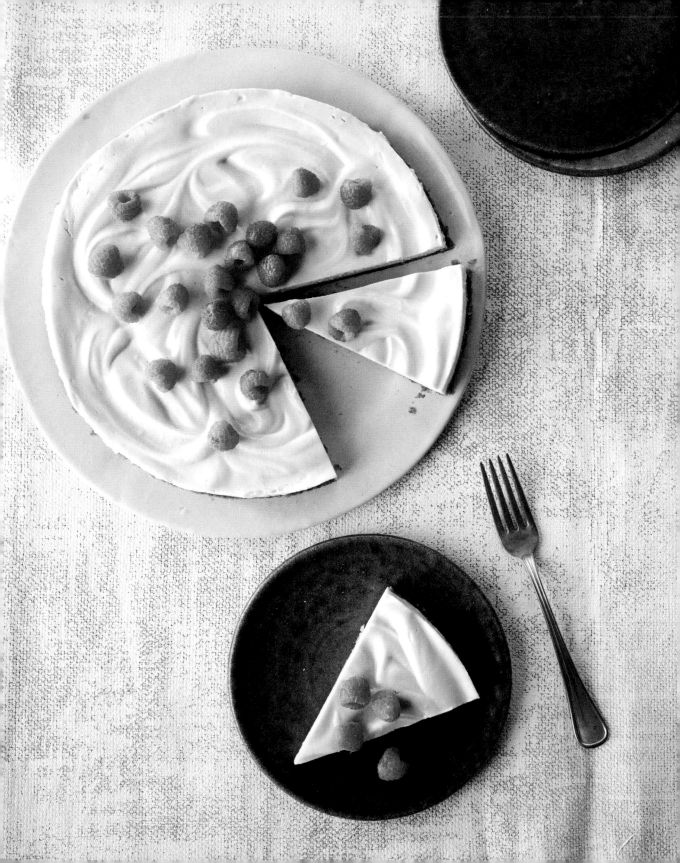

sweet treats

The sweetest part of this detox-friendly lifestyle is that you can have your cake and eat it, too—while still working toward your health goals. The following recipes are all naturally sweetened and loaded with nutrient-dense ingredients, but they taste just as decadent as their refined sugar counterparts. Though these natural sugars are technically digested best on an empty stomach, most people can enjoy these upgraded treats after a nutritious meal and continue to see fantastic results. Now, that's something to celebrate!

dark chocolate pudding

STARCH OR FRESH FRUIT | GF DF SF EF V | *Serves 4 to 6*

When I first started making the transition to a healthier lifestyle, I didn't care much for avocados, so this chocolate pudding was my solution for adding them to my diet while camouflaging the flavor. Avocados are loaded with healthy fats, fiber, and potassium (even more than bananas!), and they provide the perfect creamy texture to this rich pudding. Because the flavor of each avocado can vary dramatically, you may need to adjust the measurements to taste on a per-batch basis.

1 cup Homemade Almond Milk (page 178)

2 ripe avocados, pitted (about 1 cup mashed)

½ cup raw cacao powder or cocoa powder

½ cup plus 2 tablespoons maple syrup

2 teaspoons vanilla extract

Pinch of sea salt

Handful of ice cubes (optional)

1. Combine the almond milk, avocados, cacao powder, maple syrup, vanilla, and salt in a high-speed blender or food processor and blend until smooth and creamy. For a cold pudding that you can serve immediately, add a handful of ice cubes to the mix, or simply place the blended pudding in the refrigerator to chill completely before serving, about 2 hours.

2. Spoon into individual bowls and serve chilled. Leftovers can be stored in an airtight container for up to 3 days when chilled.

VARIATION: *If you can still detect a hint of avocado flavor in this dark chocolate pudding, try adding 1 cup of frozen cherries to the mix, which not only enhance the flavor and texture, but also create an ice-cold treat in just a matter of minutes!*

make it sugar-free Replace the maple syrup with stevia, to taste.

almond butter freezer fudge

NUT/SEED/DRIED FRUIT | GF DF SF EF | *Makes 24 pieces*

There's a good reason why this buttery fudge is one of the most popular recipes on my website. Calling for just four all-natural ingredients, it can be whipped together in minutes with no special equipment and tastes downright sinful. The key to its firm texture and buttery flavor is the combination of coconut oil and salt, so don't be tempted to skimp on these two crucial ingredients. If your family prefers more or less sweetness, feel free to adjust the amount of honey to suit your taste.

1½ cups Raw Almond Butter (page 179), at room temperature

6 tablespoons melted coconut oil

3 tablespoons raw honey

¾ teaspoon sea salt

1. Line a standard loaf pan with parchment paper.

2. Stir together all of the ingredients until completely smooth, then pour into the lined loaf pan. Smooth the top with a spatula, then place in the freezer to set until firm, about 1 hour. For a softer texture, store the fudge in the refrigerator, instead.

3. Cut into small squares and serve chilled, as these buttery treats will melt quickly at room temperature. Store in an airtight container in the refrigerator for 2 weeks or in the freezer for up to 2 months.

NOTE: *If you don't care for the taste of coconut oil, try using grass-fed butter instead, which will provide a healthy dose of vitamins and antioxidants.*

make it sugar-free Replace the honey with stevia, to taste.

make it vegan Replace the honey with maple syrup.

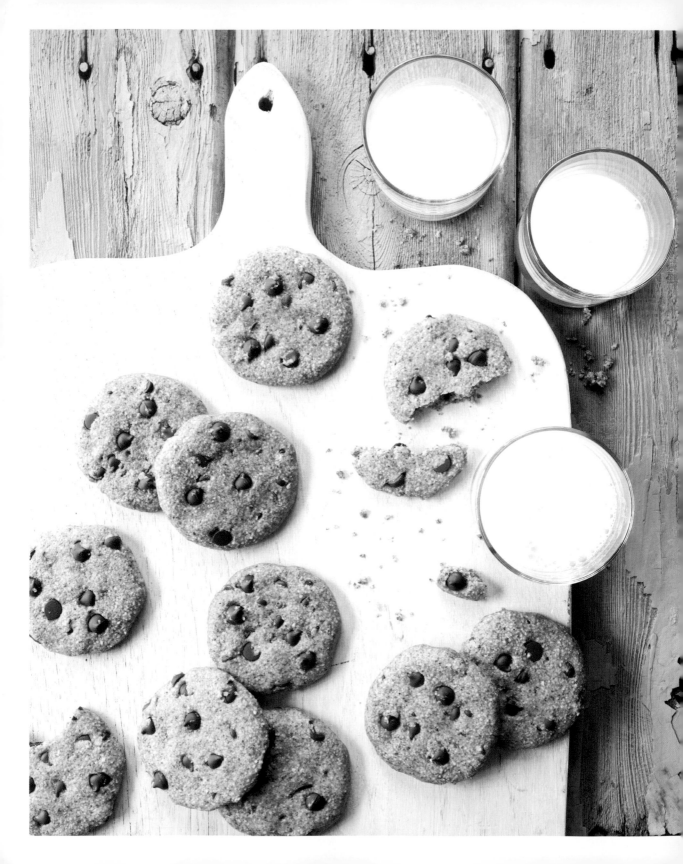

nutty chocolate chip cookies

NUT/SEED/DRIED FRUIT | (GF) (DF) (SF) (EF) (V) | *Makes 2 dozen cookies*

Every household needs a classic chocolate chip cookie recipe, and this one is my favorite. Featuring a simple base of ground almonds, maple syrup, and coconut oil, these cookies pack a healthy dose of protein and fiber with each bite. Please note that this recipe calls for almond meal, which is made from ground whole almonds including their skins, and it bakes differently than blanched almond flour, which is made from almonds ground without their skins. I prefer the tender texture that almond meal lends to the center of these cookies, but if you'd prefer to use Blanched Almond Flour (page 173), the result will resemble more of a chocolate chip shortbread cookie instead.

3 ½ cups Almond Meal (page 173)

½ teaspoon sea salt

½ teaspoon baking soda

⅓ cup melted coconut oil

2 tablespoons water

6 tablespoons maple syrup, at room temperature

1 tablespoon vanilla extract

1 cup dark chocolate chips

1. Preheat the oven to 250°F and line a baking sheet with parchment paper or a silicone liner.

2. In a large bowl, whisk together the almond meal, salt, and baking soda, then add in the coconut oil, water, maple syrup, and vanilla. Stir well to create a sticky batter and then fold in the chocolate chips.

3. Drop the dough by rounded tablespoons onto the lined baking sheet and then flatten the cookies using your fingers or a fork. (They will not rise or spread much with baking, so shape them the way you'd like them to turn out.)

4. Bake for 30 minutes, then remove the baking sheet from the oven and allow the cookies to cool for 10 minutes before removing them from the pan. Serve warm or let cool completely on a wire rack before storing in a sealed container.

NOTE: *Be sure to select a brand of dark chocolate chips that is free of animal products, such as Enjoy Life. These cookies are baked at a lower temperature than usual to reduce the formation of acrylamide, a carcinogen that forms in a variety of foods, including almonds, when heated at high temperatures (see page 22). The lower temperature prevents browning, which is a sign of acrylamide formation, so don't be surprised by their pale color.*

make it raw Since there's no raw egg in this recipe, you can enjoy this cookie dough without worry. If you'd prefer to skip the oven completely, simply roll this dough into balls and then place them in the freezer for quick and easy cookie dough bites. They make a great addition to Banana Soft Serve (page 162), too!

raw lemon bars

NUT/SEED/DRIED FRUIT | GF DF SF EF V | *Makes 16 bars*

These lemon bars are a refreshing no-bake treat that can be whipped up in just a matter of minutes. Though lemons are acidic in flavor, they are thought to be alkalizing inside the body, helping restore the body's pH, while also providing a hefty dose of vitamin C. Because these bars are made with coconut oil, they will melt quickly at room temperature, so be sure to serve them directly from the freezer for best texture.

CRUST

1 cup shredded
  unsweetened coconut

½ cup raw pecan halves

6 soft Medjool dates,
  pitted

1 tablespoon melted
  coconut oil

¼ teaspoon sea salt

FILLING

¾ cup raw cashews,
  soaked for up to 2 hours,
  drained well, and rinsed
  (see page 28)

⅔ cup maple syrup

½ cup freshly squeezed
  lemon juice

¼ cup melted coconut oil

Coconut flour, for dusting
  (optional)

1. Line a 9-inch square baking dish with parchment paper and set aside.

2. Prepare the crust: In a large food processor fitted with an "S" blade, combine the coconut, pecans, dates, coconut oil, and salt and process until a uniform dough is formed. It should stick together when pressed between your fingers. Transfer the dough to the lined baking dish and use your hands to firmly press it evenly into the bottom, forming a crust. Set aside.

3. Prepare the filling: Combine the cashews, maple syrup, lemon juice, and coconut oil in a high-speed blender and blend until completely smooth, stopping to scrape down the blender several times if necessary. Pour the filling over the crust and place the dish on a level surface in the freezer to set until firm, 4 to 6 hours.

4. Slice into bars, dust with coconut flour, and serve directly from the freezer.

NOTE: *Coconut oil lends a slight coconut flavor to these bars, so if you don't care for its taste, try using high-quality butter instead, which also solidifies when chilled.*

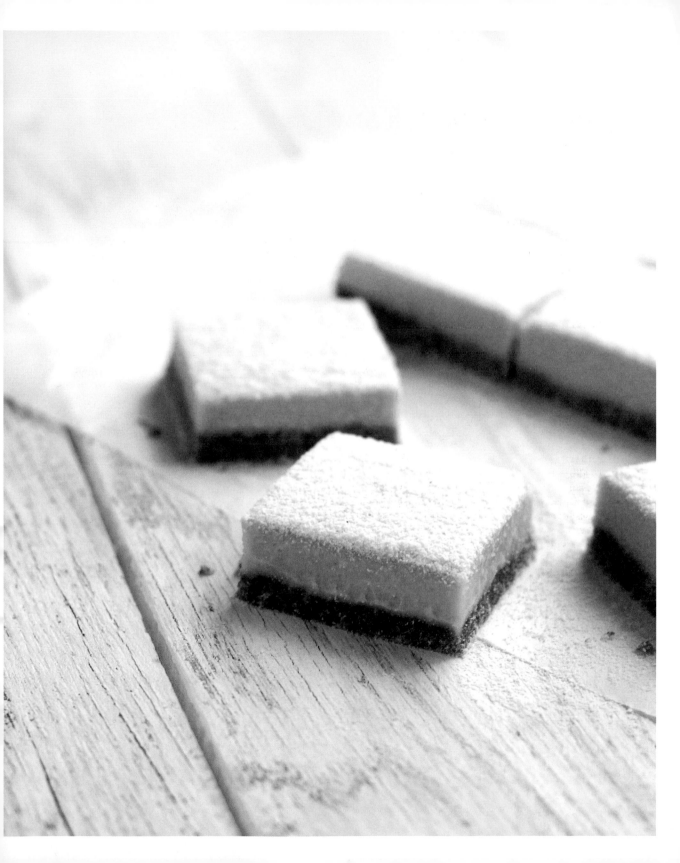

double chocolate brownies

These brownies are the perfect treat for those transitioning away from mainstream desserts. They taste just like traditional brownies, without the use of white flour or excess sugar. Coconut flour has a tendency to create dry baked goods, but these brownies are guaranteed to turn out rich and fudgy every time.

½ cup cocoa powder

½ cup coconut flour

½ teaspoon sea salt

1 cup maple syrup

½ cup melted coconut oil

4 eggs, at room temperature

1 teaspoon vanilla extract

1 cup dark chocolate chips

1. Preheat the oven to 350°F and line a 9-inch square baking dish with parchment paper.

2. In a large bowl, whisk together the cocoa powder, coconut flour, and salt to break up any clumps, then add the maple syrup, melted coconut oil, eggs, and vanilla. Whisk well to create a smooth and uniform batter and then stir in the chocolate chips.

3. Pour the batter into the prepared baking dish and smooth the top with a spatula. Place the dish in the preheated oven to bake for 30 to 35 minutes, until the center is firm.

4. Allow the brownies to cool completely before cutting and serving, as they are more fragile when fresh from the oven. Store in an airtight container to prevent them from drying out.

NOTE: *The sugar in this recipe can vary depending on the type of dark chocolate chips used. I prefer to use dark chocolate chips with at least 70 percent cacao when serving friends and family, and especially children with picky taste buds, but if you want to reduce the sugar content, you can use unsweetened baking chocolate instead or skip the addition of chocolate chips altogether. To keep the brownies dairy-free, be sure to choose a brand of chocolate chips that meets this requirement.*

cozy hot chocolate

NEUTRAL | (GF) (DF) (SF) (EF) (V) | *Serves 2*

This hot chocolate is a delicious way to unwind in the evening and is neutral enough to be digested easily after any meal. Made with homemade almond milk, raw cacao powder, and pure maple syrup, this recipe packs a healthy dose of antioxidants with each sip and can be prepared in just a matter of minutes on the stove.

2 cups Homemade Almond Milk (page 178)

2 tablespoons raw cacao powder or cocoa powder

2 tablespoons maple syrup

1 teaspoon vanilla extract

1. In a small saucepan over medium-high heat, whisk together the almond milk, cacao powder, maple syrup, and vanilla, breaking up any clumps.

2. Once the mixture is warm, but not boiling, pour into two mugs and serve immediately.

make it sugar-free Omit the maple syrup and use stevia, to taste.

strawberry lime sorbet

FRESH FRUIT | GF DF NF SF EF V | *Serves 4 to 6*

You're just minutes away from enjoying a refreshing sorbet that tastes just as delicious as one you'd find at an ice cream shop. Frozen strawberries, whose red flesh contains a compound that may help promote fat loss and boost short-term memory, are the key to this delectable treat, as they provide a slushy, sorbetlike texture when pureed. No need for an ice cream maker! Once you get the hang of it, feel free to use any other frozen fruit you like for an endless number of flavor possibilities.

1 pound frozen strawberries

2 tablespoons freshly squeezed lime juice

¼ cup maple syrup

¼ cup water, or more as needed to facilitate blending

In a large food processor fitted with an "S" blade, combine the strawberries, lime juice, maple syrup, and water. Process until the strawberries are completely broken down, which may take several minutes, creating a smooth and thick consistency similar to sorbet. Add more water, if needed, to achieve this smooth texture, and then serve immediately.

NOTE: *Leftovers can be stored in a sealed container in the freezer, but they will become rock hard when frozen. To serve again, remove from the freezer and thaw for 20 to 30 minutes, until the sorbet can be stirred and restored to its original texture.*

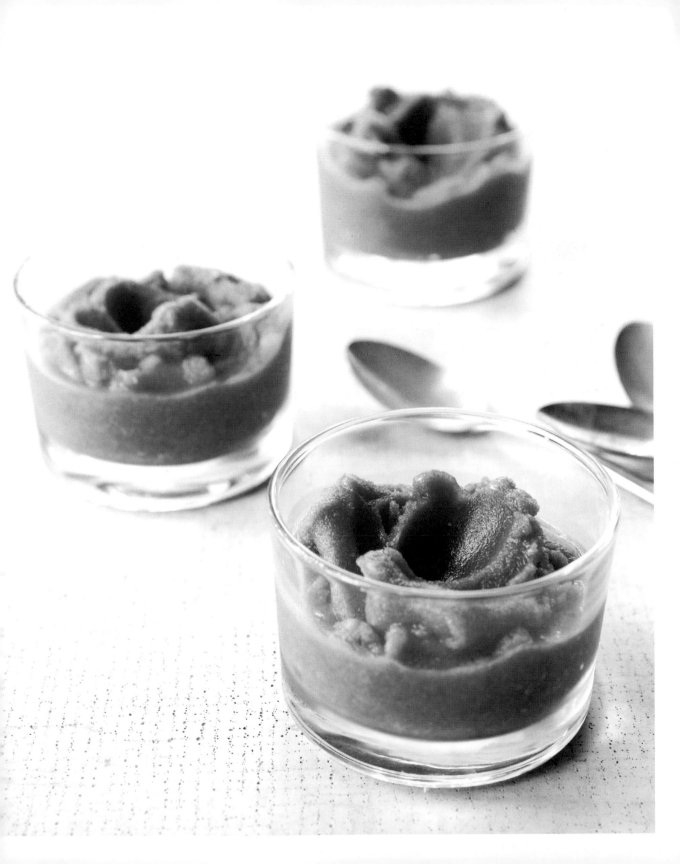

no-bake chocolate macaroons

NUT/SEED/DRIED FRUIT | (GF) (DF) (SF) (EF) (V) | *Makes 20 pieces*

These chocolaty coconut mounds are reminiscent of the popular no-bake cookies made with peanut butter and oats, but they're even better because they're easier to digest and faster to prepare. Fiber-rich almond butter acts as a natural binder in these cookies, so there's no need for flour or excess sugar. Serve and store directly from the freezer for the best texture and don't be surprised if these naturally sweetened treats disappear before your eyes—they're quite addictive!

2 cups shredded
   unsweetened coconut
½ cup raw cacao powder
½ cup maple syrup
¼ cup Raw Almond Butter
   (page 179)
¼ teaspoon sea salt

1. Line a plate with parchment paper.

2. Place all of the ingredients in a large mixing bowl and stir well to combine, until a sticky dough has formed.

3. Use a tablespoon to scoop the dough, then drop by mounds onto the prepared plate. Use your fingers to shape the cookies, if necessary, and repeat with the remaining dough.

4. Place in the freezer to set for at least 1 hour, then serve chilled. Store in an airtight container in the freezer for up to 2 months.

chocolate cupcakes

SPECIAL TREAT | (GF) (DF) (NF) (SF) | *Makes 12 cupcakes*

These chocolate cupcakes are grain-free, naturally sweetened, and feature an irresistibly classic chocolate flavor. Don't be concerned about the small amount of coconut flour called for in this recipe—it isn't a typo. Coconut flour is incredibly absorbent and just a small amount creates a fluffy, cakelike texture when paired with plenty of protein-rich eggs. Top them off with a spoonful of Chocolate Avocado Buttercream (page 160) for totally decadent, and secretly healthier, party treats.

½ cup coconut flour

½ cup cocoa powder

½ teaspoon baking soda

½ teaspoon sea salt

6 eggs, at room temperature

½ cup melted coconut oil

¼ cup water

¾ cup maple syrup, at room temperature

2 teaspoons vanilla extract

1. Preheat the oven to 350°F and line a standard 12-cup muffin tin with parchment or silicone baking cups.

2. In a large mixing bowl, whisk together the coconut flour, cocoa powder, baking soda, and salt, breaking up any clumps. Add the eggs, coconut oil, maple syrup, and vanilla and mix well to create a uniform batter.

3. Spoon the batter into the baking cups and bake until the centers feel firm to a light touch, 22 to 25 minutes. Cool completely, then top with your favorite buttercream.

NOTE: *These cupcakes do not adhere to strict food-combining rules, as they combine coconut flour with eggs, but they are the perfect upgrade for those transitioning away from traditional baked goods filled with refined flour and sugar. Remember, there's no need to be militant when it comes to how you eat—it's what you do most of the time that counts.*

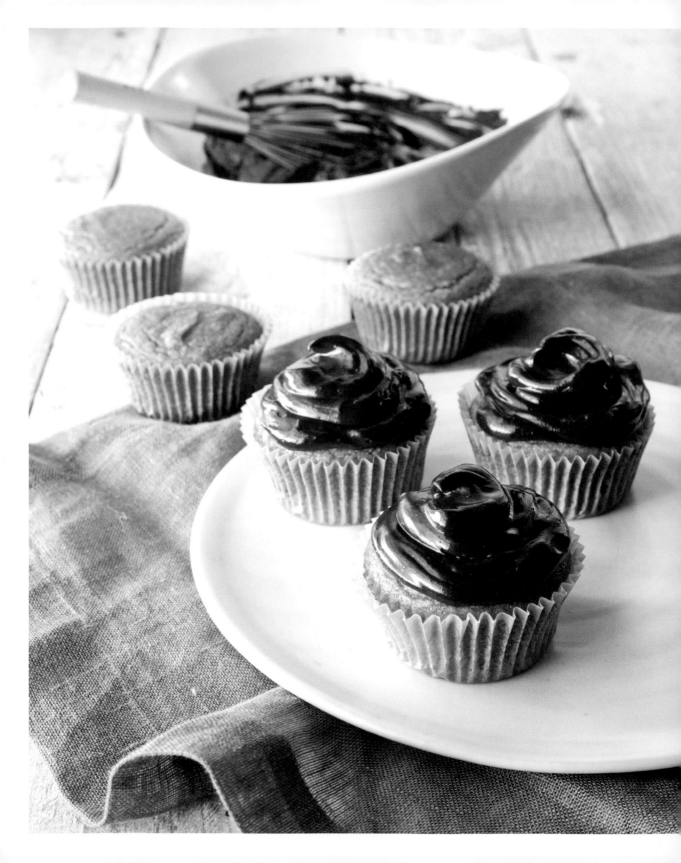

very vanilla cupcakes

SPECIAL TREAT | GF DF NF SF | *Makes 12 cupcakes*

These grain-free cupcakes are loaded with protein and fiber, but they have the taste and texture of a traditional yellow cupcake. Healthy fats and proteins work together in this recipe to help prevent insulin spikes, while pure maple syrup lends its natural sweetness to these cupcakes, along with minerals like iron, calcium, and zinc. I recommend using room-temperature ingredients to help keep this batter smooth and thin, like traditional cake batter, but don't be discouraged if your batter becomes thick from using chilled ingredients—the resulting cupcakes will turn out well regardless!

¾ cup coconut flour

6 eggs, at room temperature

⅓ cup melted coconut oil

¼ cup water

¾ cup maple syrup

2 tablespoons vanilla extract

1 teaspoon baking soda

1. Preheat the oven to 350°F and line a standard 12-cup muffin tin with parchment or silicone baking cups.

2. In a large bowl, whisk together all of the ingredients until a uniform batter is created and no clumps remain.

3. Spoon the batter into the baking cups and bake until the centers are firm, 20 to 23 minutes. Let the cupcakes cool in the pan for 10 minutes, then transfer to a wire rack to cool completely. Frost with Maple Buttercream (page 161) or Chocolate Avocado Buttercream (pictured; page 160) for a decadent treat that is sure to impress.

NOTE: Unlike almond flour, which can be easily made at home (see page 173), I recommend using store-bought coconut flour for best results in these grain-free baked goods.

If you'd prefer to skip the added oil, unsweetened applesauce can be substituted with similar results.

chocolate avocado buttercream

STARCH | GF DF NF SF EF V | *Makes 2 ½ cups (enough to generously frost 12 cupcakes)*

This rich chocolate frosting gets its buttery texture from one of the healthiest foods on the planet—a ripe avocado! Avocados contain a variety of essential nutrients, along with fiber, protein, and phytochemicals that may help reduce inflammation in the body. Be sure to use a good blender when making this frosting, as it is essential for the coconut oil to be emulsified with the avocado for a silky-smooth topping that can be served at room temperature. (Pictured on page 158.)

1 ripe avocado, pitted
 (about ½ cup mashed)

1 cup raw cacao powder
 or cocoa powder

1 cup maple syrup

½ cup melted coconut oil

½ teaspoon vanilla extract

⅛ teaspoon sea salt

1. Combine all of the ingredients in a high-speed blender and blend until completely smooth and creamy. If there are any clumps, be sure to keep blending until the mixture is slightly warm and silky-smooth.

2. Depending on the texture you desire, you can use this buttercream right away or place it in the refrigerator to chill for a thicker and firmer frosting. This buttercream will become quite firm and almost fudgelike when chilled, but it will soften again when brought to room temperature. Store any extra frosting in the fridge for a fudgy treat that's delicious on its own.

maple buttercream

STARCH | (GF) (DF) (NF) (SF) (EF) (V) | *Makes 2 cups (enough to generously frost 12 cupcakes)*

This frosting gets its thick texture from an unexpected source: sweet potatoes! Depending on the color you'd like your buttercream to be, feel free to use sweet potatoes with orange or white flesh, as both provide delicious results. Serve on top of vanilla or chocolate cupcakes for a rich, maple-flavored treat.

1 cup steamed and mashed sweet potato, peeled (about 1 large sweet potato)

½ cup melted coconut oil

½ cup maple syrup

2 teaspoons vanilla extract

⅛ teaspoon sea salt

1. While the sweet potatoes are still slightly warm, combine all of the ingredients in a blender and blend until completely smooth.

2. Allow the buttercream to chill in the refrigerator for at least 2 hours, and then stir well before decorating your favorite cake or cupcakes.

banana soft serve

FRESH FRUIT | GF DF NF SF EF V | *Serves 4*

This is the easiest and healthiest ice cream on the planet. All you need is a food processor or blender along with a few frozen bananas to make this naturally sweetened and dairy-free treat. What I love about this recipe is that it is highly adaptable and absolutely foolproof. If you want to hide the banana flavor, feel free to add in a spoonful of cocoa powder for a chocolate variation (pictured here), or throw in some raw cookie dough bites (see page 149) for a decadent cookie dough ice cream. Let your creativity go wild!

4 frozen bananas

2 to 4 tablespoons water, as needed to facilitate blending

In a large food processor fitted with an "S" blade, combine the frozen bananas and 2 tablespoons of the water and process until the mixture has a smooth and creamy texture that resembles soft serve ice cream. Add more water, if necessary, to facilitate blending. Serve immediately.

NOTE: *To make this process even easier, peel and slice your bananas into small coins before freezing. Smaller pieces mean less work for your machine, so your ice cream will be ready to eat in no time!*

Bananas are an exception to the "eat fruit alone" rule, so you can enjoy this simple dessert after a raw nut–based meal, like the Creamy Caesar Salad (page 81), or after a salad topped with fresh avocado, if you like.

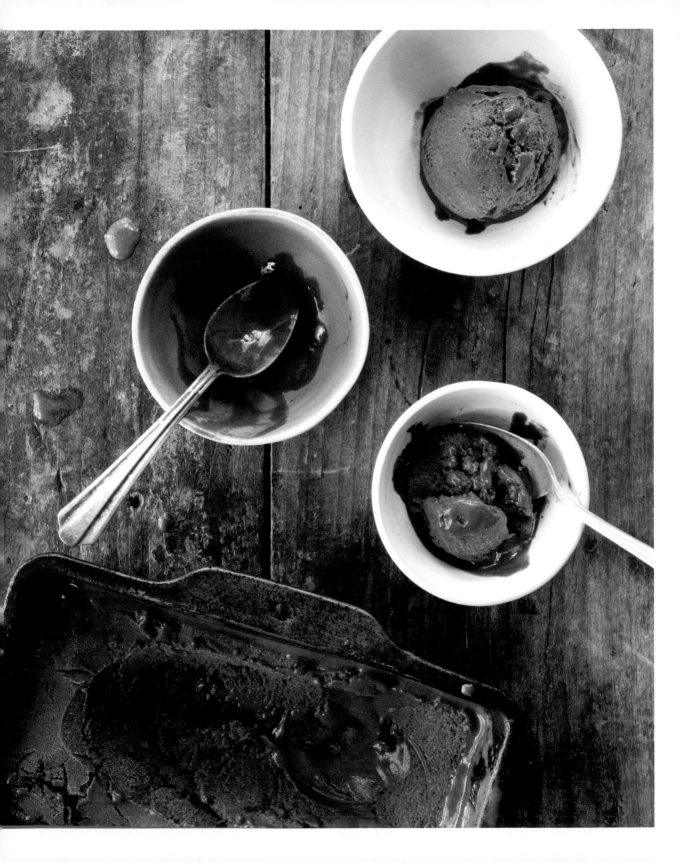

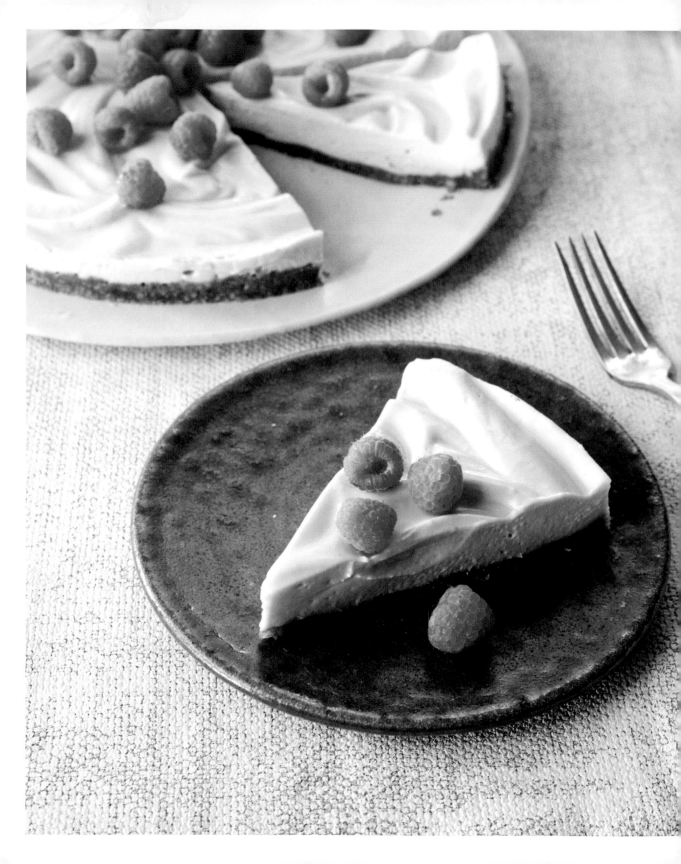

raw cheesecake

NUT/SEED/DRIED FRUIT | GF DF SF EF | *Serves 16*

This cheesecake is one of my favorite desserts to serve to those who are resistant to trying "healthy" food. It has a taste and texture remarkably similar to the real thing, without the need for dairy, flour, or refined sugar. A sneaky serving of zucchini blends seamlessly into this creamy dessert, and when paired with raw cashews, it packs a healthy dose of magnesium, which helps lower blood pressure, relieve muscle tension, and promote healthy bones. For best texture, serve this cheesecake chilled, as it will soften quickly at room temperature.

CRUST

1½ cups raw pecan or walnut halves

2 tablespoons maple syrup

2 tablespoons melted coconut oil

⅛ teaspoon sea salt

FILLING

2 cups raw cashews, soaked for 2 hours, drained well, and rinsed (see page 28)

1 cup peeled and diced zucchini

3 tablespoons freshly squeezed lemon juice

¼ cup melted coconut oil

½ cup honey

1 teaspoon vanilla extract

¼ teaspoon sea salt

1. Line a 9-inch springform pan or 9-inch square baking dish with parchment paper for easy removal.

2. Prepare the crust: In a large food processor fitted with an "S" blade, pulse the nuts until they are finely ground. (Be careful not to overprocess, as you don't want them to release their oils and become nut butter.) Add the syrup, coconut oil, and salt and process again to combine. Press the mixture evenly into the bottom of the lined pan and place in the freezer to set while you prepare the filling.

3. Prepare the filling: In a high-speed blender, blend the cashews until finely ground. (It's okay if they start to turn into cashew butter.) Add in the diced zucchini, lemon juice, coconut oil, honey, vanilla, and salt and blend again until completely smooth and creamy. You may need to stop and scrape down the blender a few times to achieve this texture.

4. Remove the crust from the freezer and pour the cheesecake filling into the pan. Use a spatula to smooth the top, and then return to the freezer to set until firm, about 6 hours. Slice and serve directly from the freezer for the best texture.

NOTE: *If you don't have access to a high-speed blender, you can replace the whole cashews in this recipe with ¾ cup prepared raw cashew butter instead.*

For a properly combined dessert, skip the fresh raspberries. If food combining isn't a big concern of yours, this fresh fruit garnish looks beautiful.

peppermint fudge bars

NUT/SEED/DRIED FRUIT | (GF) (DF) (SF) (EF) (V) | *Makes 25 bars*

These rich bars are a decadent no-bake treat that reminds me of my favorite minty Girl Scout cookies. Featuring coconut oil, which has anti-inflammatory and antibacterial properties, along with raw cacao powder, a satisfying source of antioxidants, magnesium, iron, and fiber, they pack a nutritional punch in each fudgy bite. This recipe is surprisingly quick and easy to prepare, but be sure to allow adequate time for your maple syrup to come to room temperature before attempting to make the filling, as cold maple syrup will cause the coconut oil to clump. If this does happen, simply place the mixture in a warm area in the kitchen until it melts again, then whisk well to create a silky-smooth filling.

CRUST

1½ cups Almond Meal (page 173)

3 tablespoons melted coconut oil

3 tablespoons maple syrup

¼ cup raw cacao powder

⅛ tsp salt

FILLING

¾ cup maple syrup, at room temperature

1 level cup raw cacao powder

½ cup melted coconut oil

¾ teaspoon pure peppermint extract

1. Line a 9-inch square baking dish with parchment paper.

2. Prepare the crust: In a medium mixing bowl, combine all of the crust ingredients and mix well to create a thick and sticky dough. Press the dough evenly into the bottom of the lined baking dish and set it aside while you prepare the filling.

3. Prepare the filling: Combine all of the filling ingredients in a medium mixing bowl and whisk them together until completely smooth, with no clumps of cacao powder remaining. Pour the filling over the prepared crust and smooth the top with a spatula. Place the pan in the freezer to chill until firm, about 30 minutes.

4. Cut into small squares and serve chilled. Store in the freezer for very firm squares or in the refrigerator for a softer mint chocolate filling.

NOTE: *To create thicker bars use a standard 9 by 5-inch loaf pan.*

spiced sweet potato pudding

STARCH | GF DF SF EF V | *Serves 4 to 6*

You can enjoy the flavors of fall year-round with this comforting sweet potato pudding. A simple blend of baked sweet potatoes, pure maple syrup, and spices, this easy dish tastes like pumpkin pie, but without all the work that goes into making it. Sweet potatoes, sometimes labeled as yams, have nearly twice as much fiber as other potatoes, and when paired with cinnamon, which may help balance glucose and cholesterol levels in the body,[1] this pudding is quite an upgrade from your average treat.

2 sweet potatoes

1 cup unsweetened Homemade Almond Milk (page 178)

6 tablespoons maple syrup

1 teaspoon ground cinnamon

½ teaspoon ground ginger

¼ teaspoon ground cloves

1. Preheat the oven to 400°F.

2. Poke the sweet potatoes with a fork several times to vent and place them on a baking sheet. Bake until tender, 45 to 60 minutes. Baking the sweet potatoes gives this pudding an irresistible caramelized flavor, but for a faster option, you could also peel and chop the sweet potatoes and steam them in a saucepot for 10 to 15 minutes, until fork-tender, if you prefer.

3. Peel and fork-mash the cooked sweet potatoes, then measure out 2 cups to use for this recipe. (If you have any leftover sweet potato, you can save it to add to a morning smoothie.) Combine the mashed sweet potato with the rest of the ingredients in a high-speed blender and blend until completely smooth. Chill the pudding for at least 2 hours before serving and store leftovers in an airtight container in the refrigerator for up to 1 week.

make it sugar free Omit the maple syrup and use stevia to taste.

chocolate pecan crumble bars

NUT/SEED/DRIED FRUIT | GF DF SF EF V | *Makes 16 bars*

These bars look as impressive as they taste, but they are deceptively easy to prepare. Featuring buttery pecans and fiber-rich dates, these bars are loaded with minerals, including magnesium, manganese, copper, and iron, and are teamed up with a homemade chocolate layer that's bursting with antioxidants. Because they are a raw, no-bake dessert, be sure to serve these bars directly from the refrigerator or freezer for best texture.

CRUST AND CRUMBLE TOPPING

3 cups raw pecan halves

8 soft Medjool dates, pitted

¼ cup melted coconut oil

½ teaspoon sea salt

CHOCOLATE FILLING

½ cup raw cacao powder or cocoa powder

¼ cup melted coconut oil

¼ cup maple syrup, at room temperature

1. Line a 9-inch square baking dish with parchment paper and set aside.

2. Prepare the crust and topping: Place the pecans in a food processor fitted with an "S" blade and process until they are ground into a meal. Add in the dates, coconut oil, and salt and process again until the dough sticks together when pressed between your fingers.

3. Reserve 1 cup of this mixture for the crumble topping and press the rest of the dough evenly into the lined baking dish, then set aside.

4. Prepare the filling: In a medium bowl, whisk together the cacao powder, coconut oil, and syrup until smooth. Pour the chocolate filling over the crust and smooth the top with a spatula.

5. Sprinkle the remaining 1 cup of crumble over the top of the chocolate layer and use your hands to gently press the topping into the chocolate filling. Place in the freezer to set for at least 2 hours and then cut into bars and serve chilled.

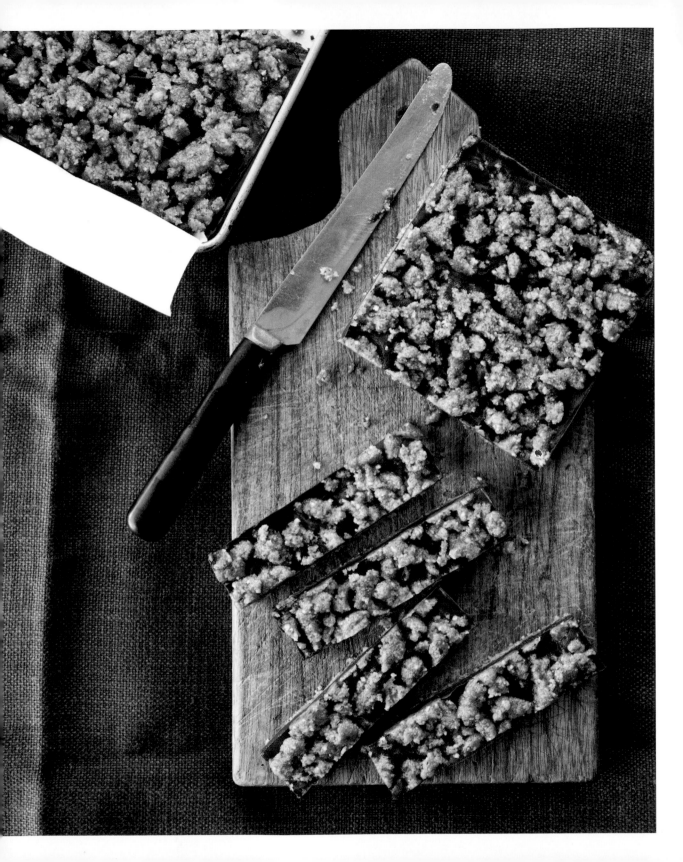

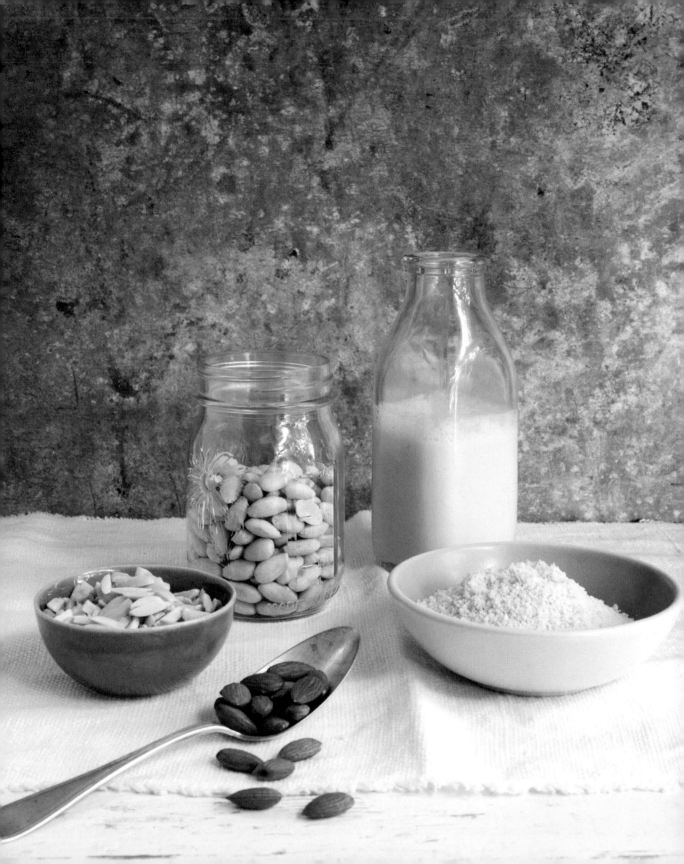

back to basics

These dairy-free and grain-free alternatives will soon become staples in your detox-friendly kitchen. While more companies are starting to cater to health-minded consumers, their packaged options often contain stabilizers and preservatives that can negatively affect their flavor and may ultimately leave you missing your old standbys. Luckily, with homemade options like Classic Coffee Creamer (page 174), Walnut "Parmesan" (page 181), and Mushroom Gravy (page 178), you can still enjoy the tastes you love, without spending a lot of time in the kitchen. Once you discover how easy and delicious these basics can be, you'll never go back!

baked spaghetti squash

NEUTRAL | GF DF NF SF NS EF V | *Serves 2 to 4*

Spaghetti squash is one of my favorite alternatives to traditional pasta, as it's naturally gluten-free and doesn't require any special equipment to create healthy spaghetti-like "noodles." Loaded with a range of vitamins and minerals, including vitamin C, folate, and manganese, spaghetti squash is a nutritious addition to any meal. With a slightly sweet and fairly neutral flavor, it will pair well with your favorite pasta sauce. Unlike most starchy winter squashes, this unique squash has a high water content that makes it neutral enough to be enjoyed with any toppings for a properly combined meal. (Pictured on page 135.)

1 (3½-pound) spaghetti squash

1. Preheat the oven to 400°F. Cut the spaghetti squash in half lengthwise, and then use a spoon to scoop out and discard the stringy center and seeds.

2. Place the squash on a rimmed baking sheet, cut side down, and bake for 45 to 60 minutes, depending on the size of the squash. It is done when the outer skin has started to develop a light brown coloring and can be easily pierced with a fork.

3. Use the tines of a fork to carefully scrape the cooked flesh, creating spaghetti noodle–like strands. Serve immediately with your favorite pasta sauce or use it in my Pantry Pad Thai (page 137) or Cheesy Jalapeño Casserole (page 118).

basic cauliflower "rice"

NEUTRAL | GF DF NF SF NS EF V | *Serves 4*

Cauliflower is an amazingly versatile vegetable and is easily transformed into "rice" with just a few pulses in a food processor. A cruciferous vegetable, cauliflower is a great source of vitamin C and also contains phytochemicals that may help protect against cancer. Although cruciferous vegetables naturally contain chemicals that may inhibit thyroid function, gently cooking this pulsed cauliflower reduces these natural substances while also creating a warm and comforting alternative to rice.

1 (2½-pound) head cauliflower, cut into florets
1 tablespoon melted coconut oil
½ cup water
½ teaspoon sea salt

1. In a large food processor fitted with an "S" blade, briefly process the cauliflower until it reaches a ricelike consistency. You may need to do this in small batches to process all of the cauliflower evenly.

2. Melt the coconut oil in a heavy saucepan or enameled Dutch oven over medium heat and add the cauliflower "rice" and water. Stir well, then cover and cook the cauliflower until tender, about 15 minutes, stirring occasionally to prevent sticking. Season with salt and serve warm.

NOTE: *Serve this cauliflower "rice" with Easy Coconut Curry (page 136) or "Beef" & Broccoli (page 131) for a light and easily digested meal.*

blanched almond flour & almond meal

NUT/SEED/DRIED FRUIT | (GF) (DF) (SF) (NS) (EF) (V) | *Makes approximately 4 cups*

Almond flour is one of my favorite alternatives for grain-free baking, because unlike other gluten-free baking options, it doesn't require additional flours or starches to work well in recipes. It also doesn't always require eggs, making recipes like my Nutty Chocolate Chip Cookies (page 149) appropriate for vegans and those with egg allergies. Even better, almond flour can be made at home, giving you control over the quality of your ingredients at a more affordable price. In most recipes, I prefer using almond meal, which includes the skin of the whole almonds and provides a more cakelike texture in baked goods, but blanched almond flour can be used to create a crispier and more visually appealing result. Both blanched almond flour and almond meal are made using the method below; the only difference is whether or not the almonds you use have their skins.

4 cups whole (for almond meal) or blanched (for almond flour) almonds

Use a large food processor fitted with an "S" blade, a high-speed blender, or a coffee grinder to grind the almonds into a fine meal, with a similar texture to flour. If using a high-speed blender or coffee grinder, process just 1 cup of almonds at a time for best results. Store the ground almond flour or almond meal in the refrigerator for up to 6 months.

NOTE: *If using a high-speed blender or coffee grinder, be careful not to overprocess the almonds, as these machines are powerful enough to create almond butter if left to blend for too long.*

classic coffee creamer

NEUTRAL | (GF) (DF) (NS) (EF) (V) | *Makes 2 cups*

If you've ever tried adding store-bought almond milk to your coffee, you know it doesn't taste very good. In fact, it pretty much ruins the whole drink! That's why I'm so excited to share this homemade coffee creamer recipe. It tastes amazing in coffee or tea and is incredibly quick and easy to prepare. Keep in mind that this creamer will stay fresh for only 1 week, so feel free to scale the amount to fit your needs. Use the leftover almond pulp to make Almond Pulp Hummus (page 86).

> ½ cup almonds, soaked overnight, drained, and rinsed well (see page 28)
> 2 cups water
> 1 tablespoon coconut oil

1. Combine all of the ingredients in a high-powered blender and blend until the almonds are completely broken down.

2. Strain through a nut milk bag and store in an airtight container in the refrigerator for up to 1 week.

VARIATION: *To make French vanilla coffee creamer, add ¼ cup of maple syrup and 1 teaspoon of vanilla extract.*

easy marinara sauce

NEUTRAL | (GF) (DF) (NF) (SF) (NS) (EF) (V) | *Makes 3 cups*

I used to be intimidated by making my own marinara sauce, until I finally gave it a shot and realized how easy it is to prepare. This simple sauce is now a staple in my home and tastes better than any version I've ever bought from the store. Making your own sauce also allows you to control all of the ingredients, particularly the amount of sugar and oil. Here I've minimized both by using a naturally sweet carrot in lieu of sugar and just a touch of healthy fat. If you enjoy marinara sauce often, feel free to make a double batch and freeze it for a future meal.

> 1 teaspoon coconut oil or butter
> ½ yellow onion, chopped
> 1 carrot, chopped
> 1 pound tomatoes, roughly chopped
> 1 cup water
> 1 clove garlic, minced
> ½ teaspoon sea salt
> 2 teaspoons dried oregano
> 1 teaspoon dried basil

1. Melt the coconut oil in a large saucepot over medium heat and sauté the onion and carrot until tender, 8 to 10 minutes.

2. Add the tomatoes, water, garlic, salt, oregano, and basil, then bring the mixture to a boil. Lower the heat and cover, allowing the sauce to simmer until the tomatoes are soft, about 20 minutes.

3. Transfer the mixture to a high-speed blender and blend until smooth. Serve warm. Leftovers can be stored in a sealed container in the refrigerator for up to 3 days.

fresh coconut milk

STARCH | **GF** **DF** **NF** **SF** **EF** **V** | *Makes 2 cups*

Coconut milk is an exotic nondairy alternative, providing a thick and creamy texture similar to that of heavy whipping cream. To create the thick type of coconut milk that typically comes in a can, all you need is a couple of fresh young Thai coconuts, which can be found at your local grocery store or Asian market. Not to be confused with a mature coconut, which has a tough brown shell, young Thai coconuts are typically sold with a shaved white exterior and feature a pointed cone at the top. If you're intimidated by opening the coconut yourself, simply ask the produce manager in your local store to do it for you—most are happy to oblige! For the best quality and flavor, look for organic coconuts whenever possible and use a high-speed blender to completely pulverize the coconut meat.

1½ cups fresh coconut water from a young Thai coconut
1 cup fresh coconut meat scraped from a young Thai coconut

Combine the coconut water and coconut meat in a high-speed blender and blend until the coconut meat is completely broken down, creating a thick and uniform milk. Use immediately or store in an airtight container in the refrigerator for up to 3 days.

NOTE: *The contents of each fresh young Thai coconut may vary, but it typically takes two coconuts to collect the amount of meat called for in this recipe. Enjoy the excess coconut water, which is loaded with antioxidants and natural electrolytes, as a hydrating postworkout drink.*

You can make coconut milk using dried coconut, too. Simply combine 1 cup of shredded unsweetened coconut with 2 cups of water, then blend and strain through a nut milk bag, as you would when making any other nut milk. The resulting coconut milk will be much thinner than canned coconut milk but will digest neutrally with any meal.

fresh enchilada sauce

NEUTRAL | GF DF NF SF NS EF V | *Makes 3 cups*

While most recipes use flour as a thickener, this gluten-free enchilada sauce uses a puree of fresh tomatoes to create a rich and satisfying sauce. Tomatoes are an excellent source of vitamins A and C and also contain the antioxidant lycopene, which has been linked to the prevention of prostate cancer. Cooking the tomatoes actually increases the amount of lycopene that can be absorbed by the body and also boosts antioxidant activity,[1] giving this sauce even more of a nutritional advantage. With only a skillet and a blender, this spicy tomato sauce can be whipped up in no time, so you'll never need to rely on the canned version again.

> 1 teaspoon coconut oil
> ½ yellow onion, chopped
> 3 cups chopped tomatoes
> ¾ cup water
> 2 teaspoons chili powder
> 1 teaspoon ground cumin
> ½ teaspoon sea salt

1. Melt the coconut oil in a skillet over medium heat. Add the onion and sauté for 5 minutes. Add the tomatoes and sauté until their liquid begins to evaporate and they become very tender, about 10 minutes.

2. Transfer the cooked vegetables to a high-speed blender and add the water, chili powder, cumin, and salt. Blend until completely smooth and adjust seasonings to taste, then use immediately or store in an airtight container in the refrigerator for up to 1 week.

hemp milk

NEUTRAL | GF DF NF SF EF V | *Makes 4 cups*

Hemp milk is the perfect nondairy alternative for those who must avoid nuts, and regardless of food allergies, it's also a great way to vary the nutrients in your diet. Hemp seeds contain all nine essential amino acids, making them a complete source of protein, and they are also loaded with essential omega-3 fatty acids, which are thought to reduce inflammation in the body. Because hemp seeds have a stronger flavor than almonds or coconut, this recipe calls for dates and vanilla to help mask their flavor and make the resulting milk taste similar to the store-bought variety, without the use of stabilizers or preservatives.

> 4 cups water
> ½ cup hemp hearts
> 4 soft Medjool dates, pitted
> 1 teaspoon vanilla extract

1. Combine all of the ingredients in a high-speed blender and blend until the hemp hearts are completely broken down. Carefully strain the mixture through a nut milk bag and discard the pulp.

2. Store the milk in a sealed container in the refrigerator for up to 1 week and shake well before each use.

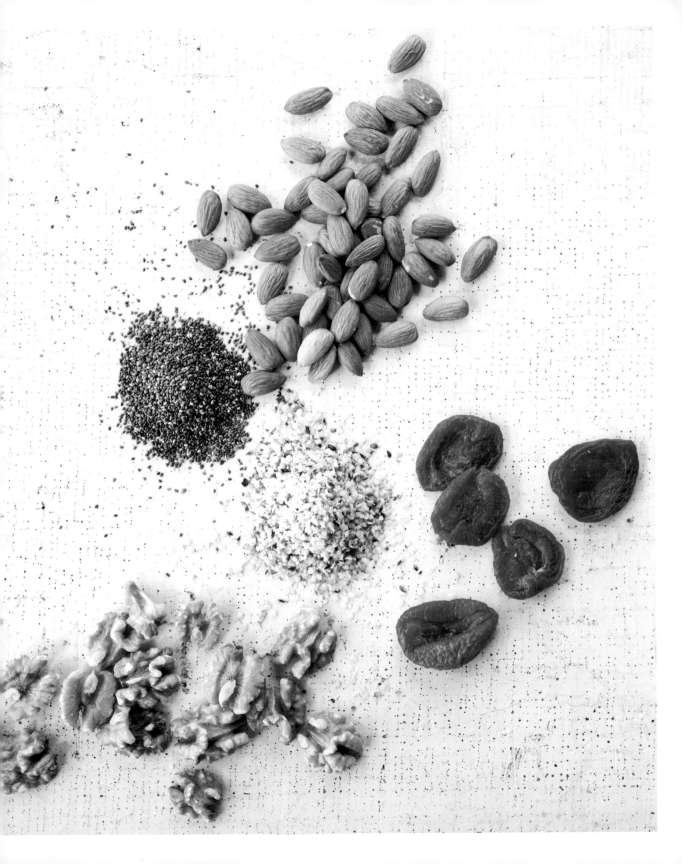

homemade almond milk

NEUTRAL | GF DF SF NS EF V | *Makes 4 cups*

This is the nondairy milk I use more often than any other, as its neutral flavor works well in a variety of recipes. Because the pulp is strained out of the milk, it can be considered neutral for digestion purposes, but it still maintains plenty of nutrition from the almonds, including their monounsaturated fats, which have been associated with a reduced risk of heart disease. Be warned: once you try this homemade almond milk, you'll never want to drink the store-bought stuff again.

> 1 cup almonds, soaked overnight, drained, and rinsed well (see page 28)
> 4 cups water

1. Combine the almonds and water in a high-powered blender and blend until the almonds are completely broken down.

2. Strain through a nut milk bag and store the milk in a sealed container in the refrigerator for up to 1 week. Natural separation may occur, so shake well before each use.

NOTE: *Use the leftover almond pulp to make Almond Pulp Hummus (page 86).*

If you use a lot of almond milk in your home, you can stretch your budget further by using a higher ratio of water to almonds. I'll often use 6 cups of water, instead of 4, to save both time and money. The resulting milk is slightly less creamy, but the flavor difference is negligible in most recipes.

mushroom gravy

NEUTRAL | GF DF NF NS EF V | *Makes 3 cups*

The meaty texture and earthy flavor of mushrooms make them hearty additions to meals and a healthy meat substitute for vegetarians. Rather than calling for flour or starches, this light gravy is thickened with a simple puree of flavorful vegetables and packs a healthy dose of vitamin D in each spoonful. When preparing this recipe, be sure to blend the cooked vegetables long enough to get a silky-smooth result. You don't want lumpy gravy! My mother, born and raised in the Midwest, has deemed this gravy "just as good as any beef gravy." So that's saying something.

> 1 tablespoon coconut oil
> 1 yellow onion, chopped
> 3 cloves garlic, minced
> 8 ounces sliced mushrooms
> 2 tablespoons tamari
> 1 cup water
> 1 tablespoon extra-virgin olive oil
> ½ teaspoon sea salt
> ¼ teaspoon freshly ground black pepper

1. Melt the coconut oil in a skillet over medium heat. Add the onion and sauté for 5 minutes. Add the garlic and sauté until fragrant, about 1 minute. Add in the mushrooms and tamari and sauté until tender, about 8 minutes more.

2. Transfer the sautéed veggies and their juices to a high-speed blender and then add the water, olive oil, salt, and pepper. Blend until completely smooth. Return the gravy to the stove to keep warm until ready to serve.

raw almond butter

NUT/SEED/DRIED FRUIT | (GF) (DF) (SF) (NS) (EF) (V) | *Makes 16 ounces*

When you delve into the world of healthier eating, one thing that may shock you is the price tag— particularly when shopping for items like raw almond butter. Although there's no getting around the fact that organic almonds are more expensive than their conventionally grown counterparts, you can save money by grinding them into creamy butter at home, without the pricey markup of the store-bought versions. All you need is a food processor and some patience.

1 pound raw organic almonds (about 3 cups)

1. In a large food processor fitted with an "S" blade, process the almonds until they are finely ground, then scrape down the bowl and continue processing. When the almonds are warm enough from the friction of the blade, they will release their natural oils and start to stick together, forming a large ball that will move around the food processor.

2. Keep processing and scraping down the sides of the bowl. It may take 20 to 25 minutes for the almonds to form what looks like a grainy almond butter, and if you continue processing for another few minutes, it will become smooth and creamy. Patience is key!

3. Store the almond butter in a sealed glass jar in the refrigerator for up to 1 month.

NOTE: *To make the process a little faster, you can warm the almonds for 20 minutes in an oven at 250°F, to release their oils faster and give your food processor a break. Whatever you do, do not use soaked almonds to make nut butter, unless they are thoroughly dried, as the extra moisture will ruin the texture. Feel free to use this method to create any other nut butters you like.*

raw tahini

NUT/SEED/DRIED FRUIT | GF DF NF SF NS EF V | *Makes 16 ounces*

Tahini is simply a paste made from sesame seeds that is often used in Middle Eastern dishes, like my Almond Pulp Hummus (page 86). Unless labeled otherwise, most store-bought tahini is made from roasted sesame seeds, which means their delicate seed oils may have been damaged in the roasting process. Instead, this recipe calls for raw sesame seeds, which have a milder flavor but still produce a smooth, creamy paste. Be sure to use hulled sesame seeds in this recipe, as unhulled sesame seeds will result in an unappealing flavor. As with making raw almond butter, all you need to make this creamy seed butter is a large food processor and a little bit of patience.

1 pound hulled raw sesame seeds (about 3 cups)

1. In a large food processor fitted with an "S" blade, process the sesame seeds until they are finely ground, then scrape down the bowl and continue processing. When the seeds are warm enough from the friction of the blade, they will release their natural oils and start to stick together, forming a large ball that will move around the food processor after 5 to 10 minutes of processing.

2. Continue to process and scrape down the bowl, as needed. It should take 15 to 20 minutes for it to become thick and creamy. Transfer the tahini to a sealed glass jar and store in the refrigerator for up to 1 month.

NOTE: *Raw tahini is typically thicker than roasted store-bought tahini, because there are no added oils. If you'd prefer a runnier consistency, or would simply like to make the process go faster, try adding a couple of tablespoons of extra-virgin olive oil during the processing.*

roasted red bell peppers

NEUTRAL | GF DF NF SF | *Makes 2 peppers*
NS EF V

Roasted red bell peppers are a flavorful addition to soups and sauces and are one of my favorite salad toppings. Sure, you can buy the jarred variety that come packed in oil, but it's even easier to roast your own at home in just a matter of minutes. Simply prepare two or more roasted peppers over the weekend and save them for easy use in recipes or salads throughout the week.

2 red bell peppers

1. Preheat the broiler. Prepare the peppers by slicing off the four sides, discarding the seeds in the center, and carefully removing the white pith with a knife.

2. Arrange the peppers cut side down on a baking sheet, and place them directly under the broiler for 10 minutes, until the skin is blackened. (The more blackened the skins, the easier they will be to peel off later.)

3. Remove the peppers from the baking sheet and place them in a glass bowl with a tight lid, which will trap the steam they release. Allow the peppers to steam in the covered bowl for 20 minutes, or until they are cool enough to handle.

4. Use your fingers to easily peel away and discard the blackened skins, then save the roasted red peppers in a sealed container in the refrigerator for up to 1 week until ready to use.

NOTE: *Try using these flavorful peppers in my Red Bell Pepper & Tomato Bisque (page 99) or Roasted Vegetable Salad with Shallot Vinaigrette (page 78).*

walnut "parmesan"

NUT/SEED/DRIED FRUIT | GF DF SF | *Makes 1 cup*
NS EF V

This dairy-free topping is a delicious alternative to Parmesan, adding a "cheesy" flavor to your favorite dishes without the lactose or casein that can cause digestive discomfort. Walnuts are a great source of fiber and omega-3 fatty acids, which are thought to promote heart health, and they may also help prevent the development of type 2 diabetes.[2] When paired with nutritional yeast, which happens to be an excellent source of protein and vitamin B complex, this topping is a healthy cheese alternative for sprinkling over any of your favorite meals.

1 cup raw walnut halves
3 tablespoons nutritional yeast
¼ teaspoon sea salt

Place the raw walnut halves, nutritional yeast, and salt in a small food processor or blender and process until the mixture reaches a crumbly, uniform texture. Sprinkle immediately over your meal and store the rest in an airtight jar in the refrigerator for up to 1 month.

NOTE: *Nutritional yeast is a deactivated yeast with a nutty, cheesy flavor. A complete source of protein, this type of yeast is not to be confused with the dry active yeast that is called for in baking recipes. Look for nutritional yeast in the supplement or spice section of your natural grocery store or find it online at Detoxinista.com/resources.*

detox-friendly entertaining menus

The following menus prove that you can still enjoy delicious, multicourse meals that are properly combined and easy to digest. Each menu has been labeled by category (such as starch, nut/seed/dried fruit, and animal protein) to take all of the guesswork out of meal planning.

BURGER NIGHT
STARCH

- Quinoa Mushroom Burgers 110
- Seasoned Sweet Potato Home Fries 92
- Honey Dijon Dressing 73

TASTE OF THE MEDITERRANEAN
NUT/SEED/DRIED FRUIT

- Mediterranean Chopped Salad 84
- Raw Falafel Wraps 106
- Almond Pulp Hummus 86

HOLIDAY CELEBRATION
ANIMAL PROTEIN

- Baked Stuffing Loaf 126
- Mushroom Gravy 178
- Cheesy Garlic & Herb Cauliflower Mash 93
- Salt & Vinegar Brussels Sprouts 91

COLD WINTER NIGHT
STARCH

- Roasted Vegetable Salad with Shallot Vinaigrette 78
- Lentil Chili 104
- Cozy Hot Chocolate 153

VEGAN COMFORT FOOD
NUT/SEED/DRIED FRUIT

- Hemp Seed Ranch 76
- Vegan Mac 'n' Cheese with Roasted Broccoli 133
- Nutty Chocolate Chip Cookies 149

MEXICAN FIESTA
STARCH

- Classic Guacamole 94
- Mexican Butternut Pilaf 119
- Enchilada Stuffed Cabbage Rolls 127

CATCH OF THE DAY
ANIMAL PROTEIN

- Creamy Asparagus Soup 103
- Maple Mustard Glazed Salmon 142
- Simple Sautéed Kale 89

DAIRY-FREE ITALIANO
NUT/SEED/DRIED FRUIT

- Creamy Caesar Salad 81
- Oil-Free Walnut Pesto Pasta 123
- Raw Cheesecake 165

KID FAVORITES
ANIMAL PROTEIN

- Broccoli Cheese Soup 101
- Italian "Meatloaf" Muffins 134
- Easy Marinara Sauce 174
- Cauliflower Flatbread Pizza 129

ASIAN FUSION
NUT/SEED/DRIED FRUIT

- Juice Pulp Sushi Rolls 113
- Thai-Style Lettuce Wraps 107
- Pantry Pad Thai 137

CHINESE TAKEOUT
ANIMAL PROTEIN

- Chinese Cabbage Salad 80
- Cauliflower Fried "Rice" 120
- "Beef" & Broccoli 131

LIGHT LUNCHEON
NUT/SEED/DRIED FRUIT

- Carrot Ginger Soup 98
- No-Fail Kale Salad 83
- Raw Lemon Bars 150

SUNDAY BRUNCH
NUT/SEED/DRIED FRUIT

- Maple Pecan Granola 54
- Homemade Almond Milk 178
- Banana Coconut Muffins 56

measurement conversion charts

VOLUME

U.S.	IMPERIAL	METRIC
1 tablespoon	½ fl oz	15 ml
2 tablespoons	1 fl oz	30 ml
¼ cup	2 fl oz	60 ml
⅓ cup	3 fl oz	90 ml
½ cup	4 fl oz	120 ml
⅔ cup	5 fl oz (¼ pint)	150 ml
¾ cup	6 fl oz	180 ml
1 cup	8 fl oz (⅓ pint)	240 ml
1¼ cups	10 fl oz (½ pint)	300 ml
2 cups (1 pint)	16 fl oz (⅔ pint)	480 ml
2½ cups	20 fl oz (1 pint)	600 ml
1 quart	32 fl oz (1⅔ pints)	1 l

LENGTH

INCH	METRIC
¼ inch	6 mm
½ inch	1.25 cm
¾ inch	2 cm
1 inch	2.5 cm
6 inches (½ foot)	15 cm
12 inches (1 foot)	30 cm

TEMPERATURE

FAHRENHEIT	CELSIUS/GAS MARK
250°F	120°C/gas mark ½
275°F	135°C/gas mark 1
300°F	150°C/gas mark 2
325°F	160°C/gas mark 3
350°F	180 or 175°C/gas mark 4
375°F	190°C/gas mark 5
400°F	200°C/gas mark 6
425°F	220°C/gas mark 7
450°F	230°C/gas mark 8
475°F	245°C/gas mark 9
500°F	260°C

WEIGHT

U.S./IMPERIAL	METRIC
½ oz	15 g
1 oz	30 g
2 oz	60 g
¼ lb	115 g
⅓ lb	150 g
½ lb	225 g
¾ lb	350 g
1 lb	450 g

resources

I rely on Amazon.com and other online retailers for ordering nonperishable goods easily and affordably. You can conveniently find all of my favorite pantry staples and kitchen tools here: Detoxinista.com/resources. Or you can search for the following items at your local retailers.

Almond Butter (Organic Raw)
Artisana
artisanafoods.com

Almonds (Organic Raw) and Almond Flour (Organic Blanched)
Nuts.com
nuts.com

Apple Cider Vinegar (Raw)
Bragg
bragg.com

Buckwheat Flour
Bob's Red Mill
bobsredmill.com

Cacao Powder (Raw)
Navitas Naturals
navitasnaturals.com

Chocolate Chips (Allergy-Free, Dark)
Enjoy Life
enjoylifefoods.com

Coconut (Shredded Unsweetened) and Coconut Flour
Let's Do…Organic
edwardandsons.com

Coconut Aminos and Coconut Vinegar (Raw)
Coconut Secret
coconutsecret.com

Coconut Meat (Frozen Raw) and Coconut Water
Exotic Superfoods
exoticsuperfoods.com

Coconut Milk (BPA-free)
Native Forest
edwardandsons.com

Coconut Oil (Extra-Virgin)
Nutiva
nutiva.com

Coconut Water (Raw)
Harmless Harvest
harmlessharvest.com

Hemp Hearts
Manitoba Harvest
manitobaharvest.com

Honey (Raw)
YS Eco Bee Farms
vitacost.com

Maple Syrup (Grade B)
Coombs Family Farms
coombsfamilyfarms.com

Nori Sheets
Emerald Cove
great-eastern-sun.com

Nutritional Yeast
Bragg
bragg.com

Olive Oil (Extra-Virgin)
Bragg
bragg.com

Sea Salt
Real Salt
realsalt.com

Sriracha
Sky Valley by Organicville
organicvillefoods.com

Stevia
NuNaturals
nunaturals.com

Tahini (Raw)
Living Tree Community Foods
livingtreecommunity.com

Tamari
San-J
san-j.com

TOOLS

Cast–Iron Cookware
Lodge
lodgemfg.com

Ceramic Bakeware
Emile Henry
emilehenry.com

Ceramic Knives
Kyocera
kyoceraadvancedceramics.com

Enameled Dutch Ovens
Le Creuset
lecreuset.com

Food Processors
KitchenAid
kitchenaid.com

High-Speed Blenders
Vitamix
vitamix.com

Juicers
Breville
breville.com

Mandoline Slicers
Benriner
amazon.com

Mini Food Choppers
Black & Decker
blackanddeckerappliances.com

Nut Milk Bags
The Raw Food World
therawfoodworld.com

Parchment Paper and Baking Cups
If You Care
ifyoucare.com

Spiralizers
Paderno
williams-sonoma.com

endnotes

CHAPTER 1

1. I. A. Lang, T. S. Galloway, A. Scarlett, W. E. Henley, M. Depledge, R. B. Wallace, and D. Melzer, "Association of Urinary Bisphenol A Concentration with Medical Disorders and Laboratory Abnormalities in Adults," *The Journal of the American Medical Association* 300, no. 11 (2008): 1303–10, 10.1001/jama.300.11.1303.

2. W. J. Meggs and K. L. Brewer, "Weight Gain Associated with Chronic Exposure to Chlorpyrifos in Rats," *Journal of Medical Toxicology* 3, no. 3 (2007): 89–93, 10.1007/BF03160916.

3. A. Navas-Acien, E. K. Silbergeld, R. Pastor-Barriuso, and E. Guallar, "Arsenic Exposure and Prevalence of Type 2 Diabetes in US Adults," *The Journal of the American Medical Association* 300, no. 7 (2008): 814–22, 10.1001/jama.300.7.814.

4. Nora T. Gedgaudas, *Primal Body, Primal Mind: Beyond the Paleo Diet for Total Health and a Longer Life* (Rochester, NY: Healing Arts Press, 2009), 56.

5. Ibid., 55.

6. Elaine Gottschall, *Breaking the Vicious Cycle: Intestinal Health through Diet* (Ontario, Canada: Kirkton Press, Ltd., 2007), 11–19.

7. Harvey and Marilyn Diamond, *Fit for Life* (New York: Grand Central Life & Style, 2010), 52.

8. Barbara J. Rolls, E. A. Rowe, E. T. Rolls, Breda Kingston, Angela Megson, and Rachel Gunary, "Variety in a Meal Enhances Food Intake in Man," *Physiology & Behavior* 26, no. 2 (1981): 215–21, http://dx.doi.org/10.1016/0031-9384(81)90014-7.

9. Gedgaudas, *Primal Body*, 197–99.

10. Joel Fuhrman, *Eat to Live: The Amazing Nutrient-Rich Program for Fast and Sustained Weight Loss* (New York: Little, Brown and Company, 2011), 143.

11. A. R. Gaby, "Adverse Effects of Dietary Fructose," *Alternative Medicine Review: A Journal of Clinical Therapeutics* 10, no. 4 (2005): 294–306.

CHAPTER 2

1. Patty W. Siri-Tarino, Qi Sun, Frank B. Hu, and Ronald M Krauss, "Meta-Analysis of Prospective Cohort Studies Evaluating the Association of Saturated Fat with Cardiovascular Disease," *American Journal of Clinical Nutrition* 91, no. 3 (2010): 535–46, http://dx.doi.org/10.3945/ajcn.2009.27725.

2. M. L. Assunção, H. S. Ferreira, A. F. dos Santos, C. R. Cabral Jr., and T. M. Florêncio, "Effects of Dietary Coconut Oil on the Biochemical and Anthropometric Profiles of Women Presenting Abdominal Obesity," *Lipids* 41, no. 7 (2009): 593–601, http://dx.doi.org/10.1007/s11745-009-3306-6.

3. D. Feskanich, W. C. Willett, M. J. Stampfer, and G. A. Colditz, "Milk, Dietary Calcium, and Bone Fractures in Women: A 12-Year Prospective Study," *American Journal of Public Health* 87, no. 6 (1997): 992–97.

4. Tariq Ahmad Masoodi and Gowhar Shafi, "Analysis of Casein Alpha S1 & S2 Proteins from Different Mammalian Species," *Bioinformation* 4, no. 9 (2010): 430–35, www.ncbi.nlm.nih.gov/pmc/articles/PMC2951635.

5. Cheryl Long and Tabitha Alterman, "Meet Real Free-Range Eggs," *Mother Earth News: The Original Guide to Living Wisely*. Last modified October/November 2007, www.motherearthnews.com/real-food/tests-reveal-healthier-eggs.aspx.

6. Maria-Isabel Covas, "Olive Oil and the Cardiovascular System," *Pharmacological Research* 55 (2007): 175–86, www.pinnaclife.com/sites/default/files/research/Elxevier_Coronary_disease.pdf.

7. American Association for Cancer Research, "Charred Meat May Increase Risk of Pancreatic Cancer," *ScienceDaily* (April 2009), www.sciencedaily.com/releases/2009/04/090421154327.htm.

8. Susan E. Swithers and Terry L. Davidson, "A Role for Sweet Taste: Calorie Predictive Relations in Energy Regulation by Rats," *Behavioral Neuroscience* 122, no. 1 (2008): 161–73, http://dx.doi.org/10.1037/0735-7044.122.1.161.

9. Alberto Rubio-Tapia, Jonas F. Ludvigsson, Tricia L Brantner, Joseph A. Murray, and James E. Everhart, "The Prevalence of Celiac Disease in the United States," *The American Journal of Gastroenterology* 107, no. 10 (2012): 1538–44, http://dx.doi.org/10.1038/ajg.2012.219.

10. J. R. Biesiekierski, E. D. Newnham, P. M. Irving, J. S. Barrett, M. Haines, J. D. Doecke, S. J. Shepherd, J. G. Muir, and P. R. Gibson, "Gluten Causes Gastrointestinal Symptoms in Subjects without Celiac Disease: A Double-Blind Randomized Placebo-Controlled Trial," *The American Journal of Gastroenterology* 106, no. 3 (2011): 508–14, http://dx.doi.org/10.1038/ajg.2010.487.

CHAPTER 3

1. L. J. Wylie, J. Kelly, S. J. Bailey, J. R. Blackwell, P. F. Skiba, P. G. Winyard, A. E. Jeukendrup, A. Vanhatalo, and A. M. Jones, "Beetroot Juice and Exercise: Pharmacodynamic and Dose-Response Relationships," *Journal of Applied Physiology* 115, no. 3 (2013): 325–36, http://dx.doi.org/10.1152/japplphysiol.00372.2013.

2. M. Siervo, J. Lara, I. Ogbonmwan, and J. C. Mathers, "Inorganic Nitrate and Beetroot Juice Supplementation Reduces Blood Pressure in Adults: A Systematic Review and Meta-Analysis," *Journal of Nutrition* 143, no. 6 (2013): 818–26, http://dx.doi.org/10.3945/jn.112.170233.

CHAPTER 4

1. Ying Rong, Li Chen, Tingting Zhu, Yadong Song, Miao Yu, Zhilei Shan, Amanda Sands, Frank B. Hu, and Liegang Liu, "Egg Consumption and Risk of Coronary Heart Disease and Stroke: Dose-Response Meta-Analysis of Prospective Cohort Studies," *British Medical Journal*, 346 (2013), http://dx.doi.org/10.1136/bmj.e8539.

2. American College of Allergy, Asthma & Immunology (ACAAI), "Tree Nut Allergy," www.acaai.org/allergist/allergies/Types/food-allergies/types/Pages/tree-nut-allergy.aspx.

CHAPTER 6

1. Catharine Paddock, "Eating Broccoli May Help Prevent Osteoarthritis," *Medical News Today* (2013), www.medicalnewstoday.com/articles/265310.

2. Y. J. Yang, S. J. Nam, G. Kong, and M. K. Kim, "A Case-Control Study on Seaweed Consumption and the Risk of Breast Cancer," *British Journal of Nutrition* 103, no. 9 (2010): 1345–53, http://dx.doi.org/10.1017/S0007114509993242.

CHAPTER 7

1. Susanna C. Larsson, Leif Bergkvist, and Alicja Wolk, "High-Fat Dairy Food and Conjugated Linoleic Acid Intakes in Relation to Colorectal Cancer Incidence in the Swedish Mammography Cohort," *American Journal of Clinical Nutrition* 82, no. 4 (2005): 894–900.

2. Magdalena Rosell, Niclas N. Håkansson, and Alicja Wolk, "Association between Dairy Food Consumption and Weight Change over 9 Years in 19,352 Perimenopausal Women," *American Journal of Clinical Nutrition* 84, no. 6 (2006): 1481–88.

CHAPTER 8

1. Alam Khan, Mahpara Safdar, Mohammad Muzaffar Ali Khan, Khan Nawaz Khattak, and Richard A. Anderson, "Cinnamon Improves Glucose and Lipids of People with Type 2 Diabetes," *Diabetes Care* 26, no. 12 (2003): 3215–18, http://dx.doi.org/10.2337/diacare.26.12.3215

CHAPTER 9

1. V. Dewanto, X. Wu, K. K. Adom, and R. H. Liu, "Thermal Processing Enhances the Nutritional Value of Tomatoes by Increasing Total Antioxidant Activity," *Journal of Agricultural and Food Chemistry* 50, no. 10 (2002): 310–14.

2. An Pan, Qi Sun, JoAnn E. Manson, Walter C. Willett, and Frank B. Hu, "Walnut Consumption Is Associated with Lower Risk of Type 2 Diabetes in Women," *Journal of Nutrition* 143, no. 4 (2013): 512–18, http://dx.doi.org/10.3945/jn.112.172171.

bibliography

Diamond, Harvey, and Marilyn Diamond. *Fit for Life*. New York: Grand Central Life & Style, 2010.

Duhigg, Charles. *The Power of Habit: Why We Do What We Do in Life and Business*. New York: Random House, 2012.

Fuhrman, Joel. *Eat to Live: The Amazing Nutrient-Rich Program for Fast and Sustained Weight Loss*. New York: Little, Brown and Company, 2011.

Gedgaudas, Nora T. *Primal Body, Primal Mind: Beyond the Paleo Diet for Total Health and a Longer Life*. Rochester, NY: Healing Arts Press, 2009.

Gottschall, Elaine. *Breaking the Vicious Cycle: Intestinal Health through Diet*. Ontario, Canada: Kirkton Press, Ltd., 2007.

Hyman, Mark. *The Blood Sugar Solution: The UltraHealthy Program for Losing Weight, Preventing Disease, and Feeling Great Now!* New York: Little, Brown and Company, 2012.

Pollan, Michael. *In Defense of Food: An Eater's Manifesto*. New York: Peguin Books, Ltd., 2008.

Rose, Natalia. *The Raw Food Detox Diet: The Five-Step Plan for Vibrant Health and Maximum Weight Loss*. New York: Regan, 2005.

Ross, Julia. *The Diet Cure: The 8-Step Program to Rebalance Your Body Chemistry and End Food Cravings, Weight Gain, and Mood Swings—Naturally*. New York: Penguin Books, Ltd., 2012.

acknowledgments

My heart is overflowing with gratitude for the talented individuals who helped me bring this book to life. They say it takes a village to raise a child, and the same goes for creating a cookbook, but to do both at the same time takes an exceptionally stellar support system.

To my agent, Steve Troha, and my editor, Julie Bennett, thank you both for your excitement about this project and for your dedication to giving it the perfect home at Ten Speed Press. I am humbled to work with such an amazing team and appreciate the support from the whole crew at the Crown Publishing Group and Penguin Random House.

Thank you to photographer Nicole Franzen, food stylist Lillian Kang, and prop stylist Christine Wolheim for bringing my recipes to life with your vibrant and engaging photographs! I also want to thank Josh Solar for taking my author headshot.

A big thank-you to Natalia Rose, for providing me with a fresh perspective on detoxing and the true measure of health food, so that none of us will ever have to worry about falling prey to a fad diet again. And to my friend and mentor, Doris Choi, thank you for inspiring me with your kitchen creativity and uniquely vegetable-centric palate. I consider myself lucky to have trained with such brilliant women.

To my readers and fans, this book wouldn't be possible without your daily visits, comments, and emails. You all help keep my creativity flowing, and I am forever grateful for each and every one of you.

To my volunteer recipe testers, thank you for bravely trying my kitchen experiments, both good and bad, and for providing such honest and thoughtful feedback. These recipes are better because of you! I couldn't have done it without the help of Matthew Saladino, Teija Cheung, Courtney and Tucker Gilmore, Heidi Gardner, Zeb Wells, Adam Clayton, Jason Berger, Morgan Cline, Sara Maples, Karen McNellis, Mike McNellis, Kristina Saladino, Heather Peters, Sarah Mann, Andrea Henry, Jen van Vlymen, Karen Tassone, Laura Sloofman, Denise Haun, Jessica Taboada, Shelly Waugh, Megan Morales, Alyssa Shrum, Susan Nee, Erika Farmer, Sarah Gillis, and Terry Roche. And a special thanks to my youngest taste testers, Charlotte, Finn, and Beckett.

To my parents, words can't thank you enough for your constant love and support. To my dad, for teaching me that I should strive for work that I love and that also provides a service to others; I am grateful to you for keeping me grounded while also helping me aim for the stars. To my mom, thank you for setting a glowing example of patience and kindness, for being an incredible mother and doting grandma, and for always being just a phone call away.

To Yasha, thank you for being a steady source of love and companionship for the past eleven years. I know I can always count on you for an enthusiastic greeting (in the form of a tail wag) and for keeping my kitchen floors clean, whether I want you to or not.

To my son, though you won't remember it, you have been by my side every step of the way, strapped snugly to my chest as I chopped hundreds of vegetables and bracing yourself every time I had to run the noisy blender (which you are now quite accustomed to). Your arrival into this world has given me even more reason to prioritize the health of our family, and you have brought more joy into our lives than I could have ever imagined. I love you, little guy!

Finally, to Austin, you are, without a doubt, the best husband, partner, and father to our child that I could have ever dreamed of. Thank you for always turning my tears into laughter, for acting as my ever-present sounding board and my (sometimes reluctant) taste tester, and for always supporting me no matter what. You make me a better person, and I am lucky that I get to spend the rest of my life with you. I love you.

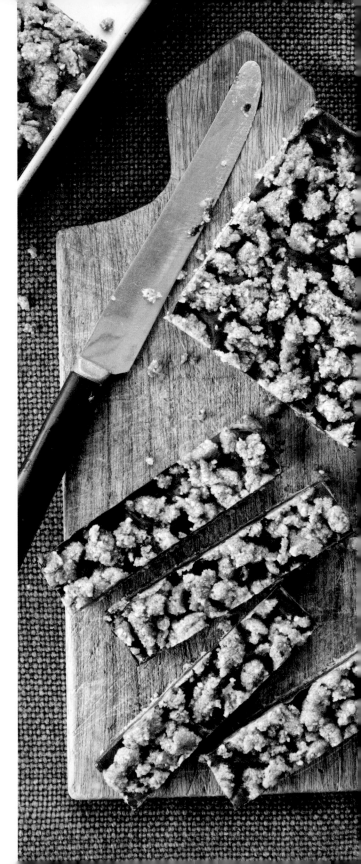

index

Copyright © 2015 by Megan Gilmore
Photographs copyright © 2015 by Nicole Franzen

Published in the United States by Ten Speed Press, an imprint of the Crown Publishing Group, a division of Random House LLC, a Penguin Random House Company, New York.
www.crownpublishing.com
www.tenspeed.com

Ten Speed Press and the Ten Speed Press colophon are registered trademarks of Random House LLC.

All photographs are by Nicole Franzen with the exception of those noted here:
    pages 135, 143, and 151 by Megan Gilmore.

Library of Congress Cataloging-in-Publication Data
Gilmore, Megan, 1983-
   Everyday detox : 100 easy recipes to remove toxins, promote gut health,
   and lose weight naturally / Megan Gilmore.
         pages cm
   Includes bibliographical references and index.
   1. Detoxification (Health)—Recipes. 2. Self-care, Health—Popular works.
   3. Weight loss—Popular works. I. Title.
   RA784.5.G55 2015
   613.2—dc23
                          2014027121

Trade Paperback ISBN: 978-1-60774-722-2
eBook ISBN: 978-1-60774-723-9

Printed in China

Design by Hope Meng
Photography assistance by Vanessa Latin
Food styling by Lillian Kang
Food styling assistance by Alicia Deal
Prop styling by Christine Wolheim
Author photo by Josh Solar

10 9 8 7 6 5 4 3 2

First Edition

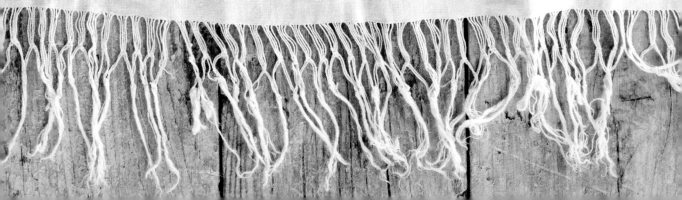